THE EMPEROR OF EDUCATION HAS NO CLOTHES.

DR ERFERT'S WONDERFUL THEORY OF EMOLUMENTALLY LUCRATIVE REGRESSIVE DISINCENTIVES

By

JOHN COSGROVE

Published by:
Chipmukapublishing
PO Box 6872
Brentwood
Essex
CM13 1ZT
United Kingdom

www.chipmunkapublishing.com

Chapter 1

The Under-Secretary for Further and Higher Education was discussing the day's business with his younger assistant.

"Have we anything for the Minister this week?" he asked as he carefully stroked his cat.

"We have to brief him on the opening of the new College of Education in Birmingham on Thursday," the young man replied.

"Yes, of course. Anything else?"

"There is the closing of the College of Education in Birmingham to be announced in the House on Friday."

"Will that not present the Minister with something of a problem?" he asked, seemingly of the cat.

"Yes, indeed. The problem is that you cannot officially close down a college until it has been officially opened. Unfortunately we sanctioned it before we realised that the birth rate was dropping so much in the Birmingham area."

"Of course. I remember the case now. Well, we must do things by the book, my boy. You will remember not to send out the staff redundancy notices before they get their first monthly pay cheques, won't you? It might lead to some awkward legal quibbles when we close them down."

"Is there anything else that needs my attention?" He asked the question without enthusiasm because the last item had tired him considerably.

"I should be obliged if you would have a word with one of our younger clerical officers, sir, Smith by name. The details are in the file on your desk."

"Very well. Give me five minutes to read through it and then send him in."

The young man who was ushered into the room was a northerner but the Department of Education and Science had decided not to hold that against him. It had its quota of colonials, immigrants and northerners.

Although he was conscious of his strong Yorkshire accent he need not have worried. The great man prided himself on his ability to put inferior people at their ease. In his younger days he had in fact been a specialist in speaking to northerners and had run courses in doing so at the Midland Hotel in Manchester attended by aspiring young civil servants who might at some stage in their careers have to do just that. He was no mere theorist either. He led forays into the streets of Manchester and demonstrated how best to approach Mancunians with the verbal equivalent of trinkets and beads. In a Manual which was much admired in the Department he had set out a list of useful expressions that would at one and the same time enable his officials to show concern for their problems and a determination not to exploit their social and cultural inferiority.

Thus it was that he slipped naturally into the Manual-Speak when he addressed the young man with broader 'A's and longer 'U's than he had learned at his public school. Although the result did not fit very well with his well modulated upper-crust accent, he himself was as pleased as Punch.

"Cum in lad. What's bin the trubble?" he asked with all the pride of an American tourist addressing a citizen of 'Worcestershire'. In the normal way any real Yorkshireman would have told him to sod off but this one was eating humble pie at least until he saw which way the wind was blowing.

"Well, sir," he stammered, "I have been reprimanded sir, and sent to you sir by my superior. He says that I don't fit in."

"That sounds very serious lad," said the Under-secretary, letting the last word roll off his tongue in his best 'trouble up at mill' manner.

"And what in particular does he object to?"

"He says that I ask too many questions and make too many suggestions."

"And do you lad?"

The Lancashire accent was wearing a bit thin now especially as he had suffered the shock of discovering that there was a subversive thinker in his employment.

"I suppose I do sir, but I genuinely thought that the suggestion box was there for me to put suggestions in, sir, and I did have a suggestion to make, sir." He faltered on the last "sir" as he groped to find the right words to explain his crime.

"Let us get one thing straight young man," interrupted the great one who was now visibly moved. He had dropped his speaking-to-the-natives manner in favour of managerial authority. "The suggestion box is not in the ordinary way a receptacle for suggestions and certainly not for suggestions from people of your rank in the service. I myself usually extend a hint to the more senior members of staff as to the nature and timing of suggestions that I might find acceptable in the fullness of time. They regard it as one of the perks of seniority to participate with me in such matters. I hope you understand that."

On receiving a zombie-like nod from the unfortunate young man he then went for the jugular. "I believe that one of your suggestions included the assertion that our mathematical experts have, as you so inelegantly expressed it, 'got their sums wrong'?" His tone, now increasingly sarcastic, blended perfectly with his accent. Smith just nodded.

"Well let me inform you that D.E.S. statisticians and mathematicians are the best, the very best. They are not wrong. Is that clear?"

"If you say so sir."

"I do say so. You must remember that this building is full of the best brains that this country can produce. Oxbridge men with first class degrees - men such as Mr Foster and myself. Have you an Oxbridge degree young man?"

"No sir, but my father has," said the hapless young man, getting redder and redder in the face.

"Indeed," said the Under-secretary, as if finding new depths in the boy. "Well you would be better taking notice of his opinions on such matters instead of formulating your own for the next year or two."

"I was repeating his opinion, sir, when I upset Mr Foster," stammered the boy.

"Just what did you say to upset him?"

"I just said that it did not seem right that the Department should be closing college after college and throwing lots of lecturers out of work when only a year ago we were expanding the colleges and building new ones at a fantastic rate. I said that the mathematicians must have got their sums wrong and that in any business venture someone would have got the sack for such a cock-up er incompetence, sir. Anyway, that is what my dad says." He added the last sentence as a desperate after-thought based upon a tardy instinct for self preservation. But the damage had already been done. In his northern backwardness he had not realised that he had pointed the finger at the Under-Secretary himself. Even the cats of men with first class Oxbridge degrees were self evidently superior and the one sitting on the great man's lap indicated its displeasure by allowing itself a half smile-half snarl. From then on it was only a question of when his transfer would come through.

"That only goes to show that neither you nor your father knows anything about predicting birth rates, wastage rates and all the many variables that make statistics difficult for people like you to understand."

The young man had by now decided that he might as well be in for a pound as for a penny and he summoned up the courage to answer back.

"My dad says that the sums are not all that difficult. He says that babies are in the world for a full five years before they need a teacher, or a full eleven years before they need a secondary teacher, or a full sixteen years before they need a sixth form teacher. My dad says that most statisticians in other walks of life would give their right arms for that sort of hard information. Yet we manage to lurch backwards and forwards every year or so as we keep getting it wrong."

Just as he was warming to his task he was rudely interrupted by the great man, not to mention the cat. They had heard too much for their comfort and took refuge in nastiness. The cat indicated to its master that it was not amused by turning its back on Smith and the great man snarled; "I suppose your father would like to come here and show us poor misguided souls how to do it then - if he could be spared from his loom in Bradford that is."

"He already works in London and he comes here sometimes," replied the boy hotly.

"Oh, really? And what pray does he devote his great brain to?"

"He is President of the National Association of Schoolteachers."

This information did not impress the cat but it did have a great effect on the Under-Secretary.

"Sit down my boy," he said. He was nothing if not forgiving to rash young men whose fathers were in positions to do him harm. "I have been hearing good things about you for some time, about your work, your enthusiasm and the interest that you take in the workings of the Department. That is what I like to see in young men - initiative and drive. I also like to move such men around so that they can get a good all round experience. How would you like to take a trip up north? As my personal assistant? I need someone to go to Dr Erfert's college. It is in the north so it must be near Yorkshire. You could combine it with a visit home."

"What sort of visit would it be, sir?"

"Well it is in connection with a letter Dr Erfert sent to us on the subject of staff emoluments. It is not so easy to understand all that he has in mind but he is a great man you know and is sure to have something of general application if we get him to explain it in greater detail. I think it will save money too."

"I have read it sir."

"Capital. Then you will have a head start."

"Frankly sir I think it is plain daft."

"Daft," repeated the great man slowly searching his brain and his Manual for the occasion when he had heard that word before. "Why should you think that?"

"Well, just look at it, sir. I see that you have it on your desk. I think you will find the cat is sitting on it. It is the work of a lunatic. Look at the title for a start:

9

'Emolumentally Lucrative Regressive Disincentives'."

"What is wrong with the title?" asked the still puzzled Mandarin. "It is obviously just a lunatic version of Hertzberg's theory of job enrichment," explained Smith, who was surprisingly well educated for someone of northern background. Getting bolder by the minute, he took the document from the cat and said; "Just listen to this; ' Put in its simplest terms, this theory postulates what many would claim to be obvious i.e. that an employer ought to reward an employee with that portion of a lucrative emolument which is more than enough to compensate for incomplete job satisfaction, yet less than sufficient to promote saturated job satisfaction in anything other than a dysfunctioning occupational environment. It follows that a gradual reduction in the relative monetary value of the disincentive by means of an increasingly disproportionate interference with the operation of the incremental continuum ought to provide so much more enrichment as it approximates to the notional national norm.'"

"What is wrong with that?" repeated the great man who did not want to reveal either his ignorance of what it meant or that fact that he had already advocated the theory to his Minister for submission to the Consultative Committee on Teachers' Salaries.

"It is rubbish," said Smith shortly.

"It cannot be," said the Under-Secretary.

"It is rubbish," insisted Smith.

"It came from Dr.Erfert," said his assistant, as if that fact alone disproved the heretic's case.

"It is rubbish," persisted Smith.

"He has got to go," thought his boss. But he said, "Why don't you go up there and explain your doubts to him yourself?"

"Haven't got any doubts," said the born-again Yorkshireman, "He is either a fake or a lunatic."

"No. I have made up my mind. This thing is so important to get right, especially as I am going to do away with the Consultative Committee on Teachers' Salaries next month, that I think you must go up there and sort it out."

And so it was that Dave Smith stepped through the Looking- Glass. Not quite in the way he expected however. For no sooner had he arrived home ready to undertake his important mission than the great man's revenge followed him in the form of a letter accepting his 'request' to take a three year sabbatical leave in order to enrol as a student teacher at Dr. Erfert's College. It was further stated that at the end of his period of training he would be posted to a new position which would make best use of his abilities. Even Dave could see through this Machiavellian plot to provoke his resignation, but having slept upon it he decided that he would not play that game. He would go to the college, enjoy a sabbatical and show up the lunatic Dr Erfert. He would then return to the D.E.S. present them with irrefutable evidence and defy them to remain inactive. This was to prove quite difficult to achieve.

Chapter 2

Dave had chosen a bad day to visit his father at the headquarters of the National Association of Schoolteachers. Marching up and down outside the building, chanting slogans and carrying banners were the office staff of that very union demanding their rights and denouncing his father as an exploiter of their labour.

"Sorry about this," said his father. "As you can see, you have caught me at a bad time. I might get lynched before the day is out. And I have to do my 'We have had a full and frank discussion' speech for the midday news in a minute. But Jim Hendrix, my assistant will see you, if you like. He knows all about Dr Erfert and the D.E.S connection."

"Right," said Dave, resignedly, as he was bundled through the chanting mob into his father's rather nice office at the top of the building. It was here, to the accompaniment of off-stage chants and yells, that he received his first introduction to the ground rules of the game.

"The first thing that you have got to remember," said Hendrix, "is that the D.E.S. is never wrong. It makes the rules and it defends its decisions, however contradictory, however perverse, however incompetent they may be, on the basis that they were right when they were made."

"Oh, I do know that much," said Dave," I do work there you know."

"Sorry. I was forgetting that you are one of them. You will recognise what we call Management by Excuses.

You may remember, or perhaps you won't, that the Electricity Boards invented it when they had a saturation advertising campaign to persuade people to buy each and every electrical appliance in sight. When the proud owners switched them on there was such a demand for electricity that the Boards could not meet the demand. So they took refuge in arguments that were sufficiently vague and dehumanised to get them off the hook. The 'cold snap had come earlier than expected' and 'was more severe than they had been led to believe'. The only people who were not to blame were themselves and it is just the same with the D.E.S. They blame their hopeless statistics on something called 'the Birth Rate' which does not behave itself. In spite of the fact that they are dealing with real live children for five years or more, they still manage to get it wrong year after year. One minute they panic because there is a shortage of teachers and the next minute they panic because they have too many. But they are not wrong in either situation. In opening and closing colleges they say they are wisely reacting to a fluid situation. One year they penalise a college for not admitting enough students, the next year they penalise it for exceeding a limited quota. But it is the college that is wrong not the D.E.S."

"Try telling that to the poor mugs who are receiving their redundancy notices next week," said Dave moodily.

"Now it is you who are forgetting that I do that every day of the week," replied Jim. "I spend a lot of my time advising colleagues on how to outwit the D.E.S and how to remain open as long as possible."

"How come a place like St.Brendan's, Erfert's place, has managed to escape then?"

"Good question," said Hendrix. "A few places can escape on the basis of excellence and public outcry, or on a geographical basis or on denominational grounds. St. Brendan's has the best reason of all."

"And what might that be?" asked Dave.

"As you know, there is a vein of pure fool's gold that runs under the Teacher Training system in this country. Your own department spent years and millions expressing its contempt for the serving teachers and then decided to put them in charge of the training of all young teachers, for instance. St. Brendan's were lucky enough to stumble upon one of the essential requisites, not only for survival in a mad world, but for emerging with an enhanced reputation."

"Yes but what was it?" demanded an impatient Dave.

"They appointed a madman as the Principal."

Dave was tremendously relieved to hear this confirmation of his own views and he sat back with a self-satisfied expression on his face. If the strongest union in the country held the same opinion as him he felt emboldened to go on with his crusade. He said as much to his friend.

"Oh, no, no, not at all," came the surprising reply.

"Nothing will happen to Erfert, and as long as Erfert remains there nothing will happen to St. Brendan's."

"Why on earth not?" exploded Dave.

"The rules of the game my boy." Dave looked puzzled so he went on. "The Teaching Game, The Education Game, The Game of Life, call it what you like. It means that you will get nowhere fast if you do not know the rules. And if you do know the rules you will not bother trying anyway."

"You know the rules and you have a strong union behind you. Are you telling me that you cannot do anything about people like Erfert?"

"Well, for a start he is one of my members and I would be supposed to fight for his job if it was on the line. Does that give you inkling into the rules of this particular game?"

"I don't see why people like me couldn't show him up and, knowing what you do, you needn't defend him too much." replied his puzzled young visitor.

"But there is more. Erfert is considered to be not a madman but a genius by your boss at the D.E.S. and by many others. Their own reputations are bound up with his. In fact many a teacher's qualifications are bound up with those of the Principal of his college and with his credibility.

"An awful lot of people have a vested interest in the Emperor being clothed. And how would someone like you attack the man? Pardon my bluntness but a two-bit clerk from the D.E.S would not get past first base, as our American friends might say. You need someone of equal stature and greater common sense and there are not so many of those around. Even if there were it would degenerate into an academic squabble in learned journals."

"But you yourself said that he was mad."

"So he is. Of course it depends upon what you mean by mad. Many a Principal is thought to be more than a little mad by the staff. Real madness is hard to detect in the world of Education because it is endemic. In the world of educational research you can get away with any old claptrap so long as it is clothed in mystifying jargon and supposedly based upon empirical findings. Some people believe that young children are best taught in huge classes. It suits your bosses because it is cheaper but they themselves pay for their own children to attend schools with small class sizes. It is all part of the game."

"Well I have read some of Erfert's stuff and he is obviously a case for a straight-jacket," insisted Dave.

"That is not in conflict with what I have just said," replied Hendrix. "Erfert may be potty but he possesses some of the essential qualifications for glory in a potty educational world. He has a German-sounding name and a doctorate. With those you can get away with murder. An undeserved reputation is immediately bestowed upon you by an undiscriminating audience of fellow crackpots and if it suits the government's constant effort to economise you can gain further legitimacy. As the government contains its fair share of loonies anyway, the two spheres can form an unbeatable combination."

"Is that the secret of Erfert's survival?"

"Erfert doesn't just survive. He flourishes. And to give him his due, he is a very nice man. Everyone likes him. He has the great ability to say the most mundane things in a mystifying jargon that convinces the audience that he must be a genius on the grounds that they cannot understand him.

Nobody is going to own up to not understanding him so they just sit there and clap. I have heard him get away with saying what amounts to stating that children tend to run in families. Then he publishes it. As you know the government is demanding that every institution produces more and more research papers, regardless of quality. Erfert tops the productivity league and, comically, the quality league as well so that any institution that employs him gets a very high research rating and extra funds. The guys who gave him those ratings are not going to suddenly turn round and find him to be a fraudster. On the contrary, he gets rave reviews, honorary degrees, visiting professorships to the States and so on. He is very nearly untouchable. Believe me."

"And do you mean to tell me that his staff and students are all taken in as well?"

"Now that you will have to find out for yourself when you get there."

"If I get there," corrected Dave.

"Oh.You will get there all right. My spies tell me that your boss will personally see to it. I am afraid that you are not exactly flavour of the month at the D.E.S. So you might as well accept the inevitable and resign yourself to exile. Maybe some of his staff and students are taken in by him but they must realise that his presence is a guarantee for remaining open. You could say that eighty jobs depend directly upon him. We have to recognise that and play the game according to the rules we have worked out with the D.E.S. The Department, on the other hand, play a much wider game with even more complex rules. They have the advantage of making up the rules in the first place, of course."

"Well I find it staggering that the world is stupid enough to let his sort get away with that sort of thing," complained Dave.

"Is it anymore zany than your mates at the D.E.S. running a system that they know nothing about? That they have never experienced themselves and would not dream of letting their children experience? They must treat it like the last colonial possession to be administered from afar as it were."

Seeing the dejected look on the young man's face he decided to cheer him up a little by confirming his view that Erfert was indeed a little madder than most in this educational Wonderland. "Some of the stories about Erfert do seem rather incredible. When he first went to St. Brendan's he was head-hunted and his arrival caused some raised eyebrows. We got a few complaints here I can tell you."

It seems that Erfert had first arrived at his new college and had lunch with some of the senior staff. The cook was put out to find that all the nice things which she had prepared were politely refused in favour of sardines on toast, which all the others felt obliged to take as well.

Over lunch he proved to be a nice, amiable man who had some strange ideas but these were put down either to nerves or to a delicious sense of humour. One such instance was when he turned to the head of the History Department and expressed his surprise that he was still using that tired old name.

"What tired old name?" asked the historian.

"Why, History," he replied.

"What name would you prefer?" asked the puzzled academic.

"Chronological Data Retrieval Services," came the reply.

There was one of those awkward silences around the table whilst his new colleagues savoured that one, although Erfert seemed oblivious to it. Then they broke out into a round of chuckles and decided that the new Principal had a deliciously dry wit.

By the time the dessert came round they were not so sure. The conversation had turned to the topic of references. Everyone agreed that they were a necessary chore. But Erfert had his own view on the matter.

"Yes indeed," he contributed, "and so unreliable. The basic problem to be overcome is that they are always written by people who know the applicant or the student quite well. Such people cannot possibly be objective about them so the reference is vitiated ab initio."

"Nice one," thought the audience. But when one of them sought to continue the wit by asking mischievously who should then write them, he replied: "If you want a subjective report you are better letting the student write one himself. For an objective report, you would of course need a total stranger. For a prediction I would employ an astrologer."

There was a roar of encouragement for his brilliance and his reputation grew apace. It was sometime later, when he actually appointed an astrologer that it dawned on people that he really did believe the nonsense that he was spouting.

"Surely he could have been stopped at that point?" asked Dave.

"Well you cannot sack people for eccentricity. Besides he had just produced his magnum opus, the thing that really made his reputation; his *Theory of Expanding Ignorance*. This was a great tome which received great reviews, including one or two in journals that he himself edited. It was based on the thesis that the more a person is taught, the more he knows. But the more he knows the more he is aware of all the things that he does not know. So, far from expanding his knowledge, a college could be said to be expanding his ignorance. The more a person learned, the more ignorant he became and mark of a really educated man was that he was able to realise and to admit his ignorance of a great many things."

"Well I can see how some people might be intrigued by that," said Dave. "It is both silly and plausible at the same time."

"Yes. And that is part of the secret of success in the world of Education. Erfert lectured on it at distinguished gatherings. It was translated into other languages. Soon he had a band of disciples. These soon split into two separate schools which quarrelled over the original intentions of the author. The Primitives took his views more or less literally and stopped teaching just short of the point at which it was supposed to induce maximum ignorance (although where that point was to be located was the subject of further learned debate in scientific journals).

"The Progressives, on the other hand, were distinguished by their insistence that 'Acknowledged Ignorance' was the sure hall-mark of the truly educated man since only a fool would claim that he had actually mastered anything. And so it was that a whole army of Erfertians set out to persuade the world that a truly educated man would always appear to be, claim to be, and would indecd be, as ignorant of as many subjects as possible."

"All that proves is that we have a bunch of nutters to contend with instead of just one," reflected Dave.

"I would not underestimate the numbers if I were you," replied Hendrix.

"They make up quite an army and are very determined. Even Erfert became marginalized to some extent, although he had turned to other things and lost interest. He never tried to adjudicate between Primitives and Progressives so, although they tend to hate each other, both sides love him. He himself got much more interested in whether examination papers could avoid the problem of being written in a language that favoured certain social groups. So he began to work on ways of eliminating inequalities. Starting with extra weightings for some pupils, he soon moved to a special examination language that was foreign to all candidates, a sort of academic Esperanto. It was a novel idea that not only eliminated harmful social distinctions but also called forth a good deal of ingenuity on the part of the examinees. He was given grants to pursue his research, research assistants to continue it, an O.B.E to recognise it and honorary degrees from at least two

21

Universities of the kind that can hide any unease behind Latin orations that effectively obscure just what is being honoured."

"You sound a little cynical yourself now," observed Dave.

"Maybe you have awakened in me a little youthful idealism that I thought had disappeared over the years," agreed Hendrix. "Maybe I do feel a little guilty about taking part in this game especially when it comes down from the clouds of theory and starts to affect real students' lives."

"You mean the students at St. Brendan's?"

"Not them in particular. They appear to be a particularly resilient lot. So are the staff. There is a particularly sane Vice- Principal called Mr Scott who keeps an eye on things. He is a sensible chap with a lot of experience and an interest in children. Rumour has it that he has a working relationship with the Principal's wife who warns him of the on-set of her husband's brain-waves. They tell me that two colleges run side by side. There is the normal, orthodox institution run by Mr Scott and there is the zany but prestigious institution presided over by Dr Erfert. The curious thing is that it is the second that saves the first."

"Won't it just get sillier though?"

"That, I am afraid, is where you touch upon a difficulty.

Things might have gone on in this way for some time if natural wastage and the rapid exodus of saner members of staff had not given the doctor the opportunity to appoint or to promote men and women dedicated to the advancement of his views and to the pursuit of either 'Enlarged' or 'Extended' Ignorance (the two rival schools used different terms for the same thing). Mr Scott managed to see to it that the advertisements were relatively respectable but he could hardly restrict the Principal's right to interview the candidates, and Erfert's method of interviewing was something to behold."

"How so?"

"Well he would have all the candidates ushered into a waiting room where he would join them and pose as one of them. Throughout what is normally a quiet, anxious, nervous time he would keep up a non-stop chatter about all sorts of bizarre topics until most of the candidates were thoroughly irritated by him. This was an illustration of his doctrine of 'Constructive Conflict' which I will tell you about some other time. Anyway, he would then launch into an attack on the college, on the Principal, and even upon the institutions to which they themselves belonged. Only a certain type of candidate could put up with this sort of barrage. The best sort tended to leave in disgust before the interview proper. Some had been known to physically assault him when he asked for a quid, a kiss, or the answer to the Irish Question. Inevitably, those who stayed tended to be as crackers as he was.

"For the formal interview he would have himself called into his office and he would interview himself for twenty minutes or more. He could ask himself some pretty tough questions when he set his mind to it, so it might take a little longer, especially if he was answering well. Sometimes he got the job and sometimes he didn't but one thing was certain; by the time that the rump of the others had got into his room he had lost interest in the questions he had set himself and so he tended to stare at them in silence for some time. When he did get around to it he asked the crucial question; he would demand to know whether they considered themselves to be ignorant or not and if not, why not? He would savour the answers very carefully and employ his own very carefully graded scale to measure the degree of ignorance advanced. The very best candidate he ever interviewed did not even know the meaning of the word 'ignorant' but the ordinary sort of interviewee invariably fell into his category of 'failed with Honours' and was advised to work a little harder on not knowing a little more."

Dave had listened to all this with growing impatience. He still could not bring himself to believe in this game business. "And do you mean to tell me," he exploded, "that the National Association of Schoolteachers knows all this and is happy to do nothing about it?"

"To put it bluntly, Dave, Yes. Erfert has altered the balance of the college all right, and it may be that some great scandal will occur that will force us to enter the lists, but until that happens it suits us not to know all that I have told you. I understand that Mr Scott timetables some of his 'team' to 'mark' members of Erfert's team and that he holds rival Academic Board meetings when the Principal cannot attend so the situation is at this moment under control. I must advise you most strongly against trying to upset the apple cart. You will not win. You will do yourself no good. And neither staff nor students will thank you for it."

Dave had a lot to learn about life. He was honest and uncomplicated. To him the situation was absurd and intolerable yet nobody was prepared to do anything about it. Well he would do something about it. If there had been any doubt about visiting the college let alone joining it, there was none now. He would do something about that situation in ways which were not yet clear but which would persuade not only the D.E.S but the wider world that the game was not worth playing anymore.

Chapter 3

Whoever is the patron saint of mad principals was definitely on Dr Erfert's side and was always willing to provide his ship with a self-righting mechanism which operated when most needed. To some extent this was because the students genuinely liked "Herr Cutt" as he was affectionately nick-named by the Liverpudlian students soon after his arrival. He was a nice man and he had their interests at heart so they were not disposed to revolt too often. He also showed a real sympathy for their genuine (and not so genuine) problems. So, although he constantly came up with disastrous schemes, ridiculous from start to finish, he himself always emerged unscathed. The students who tried to better him usually ended up believing that he was protected by the supernatural.

On the very day that Dave was speaking to Hendrix in his father's office Dr Erfert was conversing with the President of the Students' Union in his own office at St.Brendan's. The student was sitting in the Principal's chair looking across the Principal's desk at Erfert who was sitting in the visitor's chair opposite. This arrangement arose out of Erfert's belief that you should always try to see the other person's point of view.

"Well now, Mr President," Erfert began, "I have called to see you today to ask you to do something for me but as you have not told me what it is you want yet I cannot see your point of view yet."

"Yes, sir," said the student who was used to this role reversal.

"If you would be good enough to explain to me what it was that you wanted to see me about I will try to absorb the issue quickly and put it back to you in a way which will assure you that I have grasped the essence of your request. You yourself can then judge it as if you were me receiving the request on your side of the desk and we should both be in a better position to solve the problem whatever it is."

"Right," said the student.

"Then, before we end this little session, we could perhaps reverse the reversed roles and do something about it, n'est-ce-pas?"

"Agreed. The problem I have brought you today and the problem that you will shortly bring to me concerns the examination system at St. Brendan's."

"What about it?"

"It is inhuman, anachronistic, degrading, divisive and distressing."

"I suppose it is when you come to think about it."

"And we would like it changed in favour of course work assessment."

He paused for a moment in this ritual trotting out of clichés half expecting to be shown the door but he was taken aback to see that Erfert, close to tears, was nodding furiously and scribbling copious notes, far more than he could have got from the brief discourse so far. He then found himself taking a back seat and his own copious notes as Erfert launched into his own reasoned argument against examinations and in favour of course work assessment.

"And what is more they are unreliable and invalid tests of achievement. Unreliable because they produce different answers and marks from different examiners at different times or the same examiners at different times or different examiners at the same time; invalid because they do not measure what they are supposed to measure. You will know the difference between 'Examination', and 'Evaluation' and 'Assessment', of course, so we need not go into all that but remember to make my point on it when we change roles. Anyway what are you going to do about it?"

Erfert was not being Machiavellian in all this. He genuinely tried to see the other person's point of view. As long as he was in the student-mode he was oblivious to all else as he relentlessly pursued all the arguments he could think of against the use of traditional examinations and he became so engrossed in his task that he produced bigger and better arguments than the President had managed to amass before he had entered the room. The trouble was that it was difficult to get him back into Principal-mode. He started formulating bigger and better demands for his own attention including one that said the Principal should sit the examination himself and then he would see what a barbaric custom it was.

Later on, as Principal, he debated on whether this was or was not a reasonable request to make of a Principal.

If it was a try-on, it certainly backfired on the students because the result of his deliberations was that he took personal control of the examinations system and announced two negative aims. The students were not to be herded like cattle (a graphic description which the President had used) into overcrowded examination rooms and they were not to be treated like criminals forbidden to speak or eat or smoke in the examinations themselves. A book of raffle tickets enabled him to achieve both these negative aims.

It was normal practice to post notices outside the Examination Hall indicating the various details such as times and seat numbers and Erfert hit upon the idea of numbering the desks by pasting upon them one half of the books of raffle tickets left over from the Christmas Fair.

Then his fertile mind thought up something to do with the other half of the book of tickets and what better use than that which they had been originally intended? The person sitting at the desk with the winning number would receive a prize. So the examination would be a memorable and pleasurable experience rather than an oppressive even traumatic one. He made it even more memorable and pleasurable by making the draw during the examination itself. Objections were then raised that the students had no choice over the numbers on their seats so he added the refinement that, instead of sitting in alphabetical order, they could choose their own seats. The problem was that, on the day of the examinations, chaos reigned supreme. There was no way of distributing or collecting the papers in any sort of order and when the first winner was announced it related to the desk of an absentee. A second draw was made but students started blundering about in attempts to change seats, cursing and swearing and threatening to lynch whoever had been stupid enough to go to Erfert in the first place. He himself smiled benignly from the front. They never complained about examinations again and they never called a sit-in in case he joined it or insisted on organising it and they never reported ill unless they were dying.

Those students who had tried it on with Erfert fared no better than had the President. Tony Green had gone to the Principal with a toothache. Whether this was real or feigned does not really matter because the Principal was so genuinely concerned that he offered to take out the offending tooth there and then. Bernard Smithson went with a feigned mystery illness which he claimed was interfering with his studies. In truth his studies were interfering with his job behind the counter at Woolworths when he was supposed to be on Teaching Practice in a local Primary School. Serving Mr Scott with a pound of mixed sweets at two o'clock on a Tuesday afternoon was the immediate cause of his illness.

Before seeing Erfert at his own request he had checked up on various symptoms in a book on rare tropical diseases. As luck would have it, Erfert, who knew nothing at that point about his moonlighting activities, had taught in the Middle East and recognised some of these symptoms. He listened intently, threw up his hands in horror from time to time and insisted that he would not sleep a wink that night unless he had done something to alleviate Smithson's distress. The student, alarmed by now, stressed that he did not want to be a burden to anybody but his protests were brushed aside and the college doctor was summoned. He knew about this particular deadly disease because he had seen it diagnosed by Dr Kildare in a programme which had taught most of the medicine that he knew. Within a very short time, Smithson was declared medically unfit for teaching and shipped out of the college lest anyone else should catch his malady.

There was one other student prank that never occurred more than once at St. Brendan's. The only one to try a hoax bomb call on Dr. Erfert more than met his match. The phone rang one day whilst Dr Erfert was happily engaged in expunging all sexist references to little girls playing with dolls or helping mummy with household chores from a well known reading book used in schools.

"Could I speak to the Principal? It's urgent," said the caller in a terrible Irish accent.

"I will see if he is available," said the secretary who answered it.

"He had better be available," said the caller in a threatening tone.

"Well, I will see for you," she answered calmly.

She dutifully informed the Principal who was tutt-tutting about Peter climbing trees whilst Jane was kissing Daddy good-bye on his way to the male-dominated world of big business. He absent-mindedly asked her to take a message or ask them to call back later. But that did not satisfy the caller.

"Tell him that he had better come to this phone pretty damn quick or people will be killed in his college," said the voice with menace. "There is a bomb in the building."

She was not so calm when she returned to the Principal and relayed this message but the great man was by this time getting quite annoyed with the obvious preference that Pet the dog was showing towards Peter in spite of the obvious affectionate nature of Jane and he was in no mood to let a little matter like a bomb scare deter him.

"Tell him to call back when I have more time," he said with some irritation.

"Could you possibly call back when he is not so busy?" she stammered into the phone.

"What are you, some kind of a nut?" shouted the would-be terrorist, who by this time was losing his Irish accent and relapsing into a more natural scouse. "Get the Principal and get him quick."

"Well I will see what I can do" she said," but he is a very determined man and he won't be very pleased"

"Oh, very well," sighed Dr Erfert when she finally got through to him that this was a matter worthy of his attention using, not the bomb argument, but the fact that the caller had been rude to her.

Erfert always reacted well if he thought someone was being badly treated, especially a lady. He took the phone and before the man could utter any more threats he said, "Look here, whoever you are, I really cannot have you ringing up here and upsetting my secretary like this. I think that the least you could do is to apologise to her at once."

"Like Hell I will," shouted the voice in exasperation.

"Don't you realise, you daft bugger, that I have phoned you to warn you that there is a bomb planted in your building and that if you do not get up off your arse someone is likely to be killed in about twenty minutes from now?"

"I am not listening to you until you apologise to my secretary," said our hero, who by now was beginning to think that he was dealing with an undesirable. Anyone who shouted at ladies and used rude language was an undesirable. The fact that he also appeared to plant bombs was useful confirmatory evidence. "Are you going to apologise or am I going to put down this phone?" he demanded.

"Oh, all right then," said the caller wearily.

"Good," said Erfert, "now that we have got that settled what is all this about a bomb?"

The man on the other end of the line perked up a bit at this invitation to return to his business. "There is a bomb in your building and it is timed to go off in twenty minutes."

"Eighteen, I think you will find," said Erfert by way of correction, "but let's not quarrel about that. Whereabouts is it?"

"Why the Hell should I tell you where it is?" demanded the voice.

"So that I can tell everyone where to stand when it goes off" replied Erfert ever so patiently.

"Aren't you going to call the police or the fire-brigade?" asked the voice hopefully.

"I don't suppose you could do that for me, could you? After all it is your bomb. You know far more about it than I do. And whilst you are doing that I could be putting up a notice in the staff room. But quite what I shall put on it I really don't know. Couldn't you give me a little clue about where you have put it? I hate being vague in notices to the staff. It is something I rather pride myself on."

"Look mate," there was a silence after these two words and then the voice went on slowly and painfully, "if I wanted to blow up the college and you with it, I wouldn't be likely to tell you where I put the bomb would I?"

"Yes I grant you that," said Erfert, always ready to see the other person's point of view, "but you were good enough to phone me in the first place and I am only really asking you to be a little more specific. May I at least ask you why you have planted this bomb here?"

"Because you represent the exploiter class and I want you to squirm along with all the other capitalist lackeys who are misleading the youth of this country."

"I suppose that you have got a point there," mused Erfert, ready as ever to see the other person's point of view. He was getting to like this caller who showed such an interest in the philosophical and sociological implications of Erfert's own work, albeit a critical one. He asked him to explain in more detail his concerns.

"If you were really interested in your students, you would blow up the whole rotten show yourself."

"Yes, I would wouldn't I?" agreed Erfert, now quite engaged in thinking up all sorts of reasons for doing just that and for assessing the professional consequences of successfully blowing up his own college.

He asked the man where would be the best place to plant a bomb in order to maximise its effect. He contributed various Marxist/Leninist arguments that left the man on the other end of the line speechless. Following a strangled cry from the voice he asked him if he was all right and if there was anything else he could oblige him with but there was a deep silence from the other end and Erfert assumed that he was either thinking very deeply or else that his money had run out. He babbled on with a few more ways of abolishing reactionary societies for enough time to elapse for the bomb to have exploded several times over, invited his caller round to tea so that they could explore the matter further, and, although he did not know it, left his new friend and would-be revolutionary, in a kiosk within sight of the college on his knees, blubbering uncontrollably, and with no further strength even to refuse.

Chapter 4.

The Under-Secretary for Further and Higher Education was tired. He had already closed two colleges that morning and it was not yet ten o'clock.

With great ingenuity he had also altered the arrangements for the Minister of State to visit a town where a by-election was due. Instead of digging a hole in which to plant a tree in a school's grounds, the Minister was to announce that he was digging the first sod in a multimillion pound extension to the school's science laboratories. He stroked his pussy cat thoughtfully and that contented creature selected a letter for him to read from the pile of correspondence which formed its comfortable nest.

Theophilus, the cat, ran a good deal of the department for him. It was a huge, black, motionless, well-fed creature and it displayed all the infuriating smugness of a cat that had 'arrived'. Not for Theophilus the worry of walking dangerous streets peopled by natural enemies; not for him the worry of scavenging for scarce food and chasing mice. Comfortably housed at the top of a luxurious tower block, it remained in the great man's office day and night and selected documents for the master to peruse.

If Theophilus did not select them they did not get read although they did get answered - with a negative. The cat had played a significant part in the government of education in this country over a number of years including the appointment and continued success of Dr Erfert. It ensured that his correspondence was always brought forward and read. The reason for this was simple. It lay in his liking for sardines and the consequent faint aroma of that

36

delicacy which always lingered on his mail long enough to seduce even an Oxbridge cat whose master had a first. Theophilus had been known to sit upon some letters for days refusing to release them until all Erfert's correspondence had been dealt with.

His assistant came in whilst the great man was reading one of these delicately scented missives from Dr Erfert.

"Do you think," he mused, "that Dr Erfert might possibly be wrong about Emolumentally Lucrative Regressive Disincentives?"

"I hardly think so. He did go to Oxford."

"Oh, I know that he is a good man. It is just that I am not sure if his theory will save us money or cost us money. What do you think?"

"I do not think that it will cost us any more than is necessary to spend in order to implement the policy."

"How much do you reckon that would be?"

"It is hard to say without going into details with him."

"Well the Minister is all for it and he is going to announce his intention of implementing it to the House next week so we need to have a figure for the estimates."

"What about two million?"

"Too round and neat. Can you refine the costings?"

"Say two million, three hundred and forty four thousand, and eight hundred and nine pounds. We can always change it a bit if Erfert gives us more detail. Maybe Smith could get some details out of him."

"Smith?"

"You may not remember but Smith was the communist northern ruffian who was causing lots of trouble in the Department until you sent him off to St. Brendan's to cool his heels."

"Oh, him. I am not having anything to do with that young thug. He has not got the background to understand a man like Erfert so it is no use relying on him. We need someone who is one of us, or failing that, one of our HMIs. The regional inspector could go and see Erfert, get some costings out of him and put in a word about Smith's being a troublemaker who ought to be fired from the college. We could then refuse to have him back here and everyone would be happy."

"Dickie Biggs-Humphreys is the regional inspector. A good chap. His brother was at All Souls and Dickie was at Winchester with me, he put up a bit of a black with the Chief Education Officer of Stockport when he did not appear to know the school leaving age but that was when he was new and he is learning all the time."

"Was that the C.E.O. who sent in that cheap complaint that Dickie had never taught in a state school?"

"Or any school, as if that mattered. Some of these C.E.O.s have a thing about experience; as if twenty years in the South African Police Force was not relevant experience."

"As a matter of interest just remind me what the school leaving age is at the moment."

"I think it is about eighteen in our set up but I am not so sure if it is the same in Stockport. I shall check and let you know."

"Right then. Dickie it is. Send him along there to consult Erfert and to get Smith sacked at the same time."

So it was that Dickie Biggs-Humphreys came to be standing at the porter's desk in the vestibule of St Brendan's, carrying his badges of office - a rolled up umbrella and a Masonic-type case. He was a tall, gaunt man with a mouth that was permanently sealed into the grimmest and straightest of grim straight lines.

"Biggs-Humphreys, HMI, he announced briskly, "to see Dr. Erfert."

"Is he expecting you sir?" Enquired the elderly porter politely.

"Biggs-Humphreys, HMI, to see Dr. Erfert immediately," he repeated in the best colonial fashion of effortless superiority.

"I will see if he can see you sir," said the patient porter.

"On the contrary. I will ensure he sees me by going straight in. Thank you my man." And with that he brushed past the porter and entered the inner sanctum.

The Principal was reading the Beano when he discovered this tall, gaunt figure staring down at him. Reluctantly he put down the comic and extended his own hand to meet and grab the stiffly proffered hand of his visitor. He asked him if he could be of any assistance.

"I should be obliged if you could answer one or two questions for me," said Biggs-Humphreys.

"Certainly, if I can," said Erfert.

"First of all could you tell me why so many of your students appear to be above the normal school leaving age - which I am reliably informed, is sixteen."

"They are all over the school leaving age here. They come here after leaving school."

"Remarkable," said the ex-policeman. "Let me warn you that I might have to report that fact to the Department. You might be depriving some local children of school age of places here. But it is on another matter that I would like your advice. Could you confirm for me the costs of implementing your theory of Emolumentally Lucrative Regressive Disincentives?"

"Certainly," said Erfert, "the theory is, of course, largely self explanatory, and will cost no more and no less than it takes to put it into operation in the most cost-effective way that can be devised."

"Yes, that sounds reasonable enough," said the Brain of Britain rather slowly. "You couldn't put a figure on it, could you?"

"Yes, to plus or minus three million pounds."

"That sounds near enough to our own carefully costed projections," he mistakenly opined. His confidence in the D.E.S Statisticians having been confirmed he thought he would ask Erfert to explain in just a little more detail the advantages of the new theory.

"It is simple enough,"said Erfert, always willing to oblige. "You understand of course that it is based upon a motivation-hygiene theory which seeks to systematise an employer's role in providing compensatory conditions for the promotion of motivated teachers. In that sense the opposite of job satisfaction is not, as one would expect, job dissatisfaction, but lack of job satisfaction."

"Yes," said the HMI already meekly bowing to a superior intelligence without showing it.

"That being so," said the unstoppable Erfert, there is a difference between not feeling happy and feeling unhappy. The hygiene factors are limited in their ability to promote the lessening of the dissatisfaction; they might be a pre-requisite to effective motivation but they are not in themselves motivating factors. Motivators are not of course the opposite of hygiene factors either. The absence of motivating factors will not necessarily cause workers to be unhappy but their presence is necessary to promote a feeling of satisfaction."

"I understand perfectly," said the mystified HMI who, like hundreds of others before him, had fallen under the spell of the High Priest of Jargon. All he wanted now was the obligatory HMI lunch, with wine, and then a nice ride in a first class rail compartment with enough time to scribble out a note to the D.E.S that Erfert obviously knew what he was talking about and that the D.E.S.'s statisticians had been remarkably accurate in their estimate of the costs involved. He had forgotten all about Dave Smith.

Chapter 5

St Brendan's College of Education nestled in a beautiful rural setting of over eighty acres of green belt and forest, just ten miles from the centre of the city. Originally the home of a gentle family, the Old Hall was now the centre of a group of modern buildings and became the hub of a college some ten years before when the D.E.S. was in one of its expansionist moods. Its idyllic setting was entirely appropriate for the Alice-in-Wonderland situation which pertained within its boundaries. In a curious sort of a way the great variety of styles of building reflected the great variety of characters who lived out their lives there. There was the original Old Hall, a manor house and a splendid example of regional domestic architecture with all the signs of additions and alterations over the centuries. There were two matching Halls of Residence, built in the days when buildings were supposed to last, massive and rather forbidding in appearance. Then there were the more modern buildings, which had won D.E.S design awards in their day, square, ugly, flat-topped and leaky.

They had originally been the brain-child of the then Secretary of State, Sir Kenneth Michael and were announced as the prototype for the most advanced system of sectionalised buildings that the world had ever known. The cynical old clerk of works at the time impressively referred to it as the R.T.F.D. system which everyone accepted as its proper title. Only his intimates knew that he privately considered it to mean the Ready-To-Fall-Down System. Even these were outdone in their ugliness by the most recent building sent down from the Architects branch of the D.E.S - the fat, bloated, eccentric, inflatable gymnasium, cheap to erect, hideous to behold.

The college proper was approached from the main road along a winding drive, attractively bordered by rhododendrons. On one side of the drive lay George's farm which had its uses in terms of supplies, casual labour and escape routes across the fields. On the other side was to be found a magnificent sports field that was to become a familiar feature of Dave's student life. Behind the sports field lay the local golf course where a good many of the staff took their recreation and where the Principal was held in great esteem. This was not because of any great prowess off the tees but because they had become conditioned to believe that he was a genius and nothing could persuade them to the contrary. The piece of evidence most adduced to prove his brilliance was his complicated and quite revolutionary system of handicapping which he would willingly explain at great length but in such an unintelligible a manner that even hard-headed business men came away thinking that he must be incredibly brilliant, largely on the basis of not being able to understand him. They did not, of course, actually adopt his system, so his reputation was not really put to the test.

At the top of the drive was a small traffic island which positively bristled with signs pointing to different buildings; the administration block, the dining room, the theatre, the library, the students' village and the various specialists rooms including the medical centre and the resident astrologer's consultation rooms. Every year a new generation of students discovered, seemingly for the first time, the wonderful prank of changing these signs around so as to mislead the unwary. They were changed around so often that they frequently ended up pointing in the right direction.

Dave was not to know all this as he walked spiritedly up the drive on his first full day in college and passed the sign that carried the old chestnut "Dyslexia Rules K.O.?" He wondered to himself how long he would last and whether the Department would ever have him back. Had he dropped in on the astrologer he might have had some warning that he would gain a few things from St. Brendan's. He would gain an education of sorts, a sense of humour of sorts, a deeper self knowledge, and a greater respect for the Principal. He also was to gain a wife and freedom from the D.E.S. but whether the resident astrologer was capable of seeing any of this is a matter of some doubt.

After general instructions and lots of form-filling the new students were expected to meet the Principal for a chat and the Deputy for an exhortation. Dave and six others were instructed to meet him in his own house in the grounds. On presenting themselves they found themselves in the presence of a genial, smiling gentleman who bore a marked resemblance to Lenin whilst the latter was painting a staircase. Two things were to be indelibly imprinted on the memory of those seven students. One was that Lenin continuously asked them questions to which they had no answers yet appeared delighted with their honest admissions of ignorance. The second was the sight of the Principal making his way up the stairs whilst holding a paint brush horizontally against the wall in such a way as to trace a zigzag pattern that exactly matched the rise of the stairs. In lesser people this might have seemed a trifle eccentric, but in Erfert, it was held by many to be an example of his brilliantly novel way of solving problems of interior design and decoration. As for Dave, it merely confirmed his opinion formed in London.

Next came a talk from the conventional Mr Scott, who explained in more orthodox but somewhat cynical terms the Teacher Training Course as it then existed, making only brief mention of the fact that the D.E.S changed it at short notice every year. "You have to remember," he said, "that somewhere, through no fault of his own, there exists some unfortunate child who is going to get you as his teacher. It is my job to see that you do him as little harm as possible. You will need three things in order to qualify as a teacher," he went on. "You will need to be of good health, of good character, and of good academic achievement. The first is in hands of the college doctor; the second embraces every failing short of a criminal offence; so it is on the third of these things that you will be judged by *me*." He paused on the last word in order to let the thinly veiled threat sink in then he went on, "you may be surprised to find that you spend only about twelve weeks of your course actually teaching in schools. That is regrettable but at least it will minimise the damage that you will be able to inflict on any particular group of pupils. For the most part your studies will be concerned with your two academic options but you will also have to study the academic theory of Education as well as some professional courses such as the teaching of Reading. You will be allocated to a personal tutor to whom you can turn for advice especially if you get into any trouble. Any questions?"

He was a kindly man but he had developed a brusque way of dealing with students which served to set the tone of their relationship with him for the rest of their stay. He tended to ask for questions in a manner which discouraged the posing of any. Dave was to discover, as were his fellow freshers, that the best way to find out about the college was to jump in at the deep end and seek advice as the occasion demanded.

The occasion came sooner than anyone anticipated. All new students had to undergo a sort of screening test to see if they could talk proper, as one cockney lad put it. Those who passed first time need not see the Elocution Lecturer again, which was a blessing known only to those released from prisoner of war camps. The others were condemned men and women, condemned to suffer under one of Erfert's most inspired appointments. He was a curious, frightening character known to the students as MacPudding. MacPudding was an enormous Scot with great glaring eyes and a black shaggy beard which quivered uncontrollably whenever he fell into one of his many rages. For some reason the object of his most violent tantrums was an inoffensive little Chinese gentleman appointed by Erfert, at the D.E.S.'s instigation, to run a course called Feminism in Ancient China. No student had been found stupid enough to enrol on this esoteric venture run by a pidgin-English-speaking oriental so he had been redeployed as an assistant to MacPudding. This led to many amusing incidents in itself but it also seemed to arouse deep emotions in MacPudding. It was difficult to work out just what was the reason for this animosity for, like the Chinese, MacPudding did not speak English in any of its more recognisable forms. It seems that Dr Erfert had read somewhere (he was always reading something somewhere) that the best English is that which is spoken in Dublin. So he tried to recruit an Irishman to the post of Elocution Lecturer. A letter of application arrived from MacPudding (or whatever his name was) who was at that time on holiday in Ireland. Erfert had appointed him by return of post on the strength of an Irish-sounding name and a Dublin postmark. The new students were startled to find MacPudding yelling some incomprehensible instructions at them seemingly to read a passage out of a book which he threw at them. The first one bold enough to try was interrupted by snorts and growls and bellows of savage intensity. Even the Scottish students failed to make out what he was shouting about. They were saved by the appearance of the little Chinaman who only had to appear to short-circuit MacPuddings wiring. The two of them put on a magnificent spectacle of belligerence reminiscent of those Hollywood cartoons which featured a growling bulldog and a chirping budgerigar. The spectacle was deficient to the extent that neither the belligerents nor the enthralled audience could actually understand the abuse that was being hurled around and so no one was in a position to score the points made, but the mere sight of the two locked in mortal combat had a sort of primitive beauty which kept those privileged to witness it completely fascinated.

So ended the first day at St. Brendan's. The evening was spent socialising and making new friends as well as swapping stories about some of the more peculiar things that they had encountered. One of the most peculiar of these happenings frightened most of them to death until they discovered that each and every one of them had received a little brown envelope which contained the same message. Dave opened his to find a note from Mr Matthew Brown to the effect that his:

ATTENDANCE/ATTITUDE/COURSE WORK had all been found to be unsatisfactory. Like a good many other new students he went racing around the college in a panic until some of the older students put him right.

It appeared that Matthew Brown was in charge of the Progress Committee (once called the Disciplinary Committee). It would be more accurate to say that Matthew Brown *was* the Progress Committee because most of the other members refused to sit with him and the Committee could not meet without him in the chair. There had to be some sort of a committee to satisfy the regulation that a student should not be failed without some sort of official warning that he or she might fail. Dr Erfert's brainwave had been to give every student an official warning at the end of the first day back thus pre-empting the claim that failure had a come as a surprise.

The students had naturally protested against this practice but they were taken aback when he actually joined the picket outside his office and offered to supply them with better ways of bringing pressure upon himself as Principal. They had dispersed, baffled, exhausted and divided, leaving him on solitary picket duty outside his own room, happily formulating written demands for his own attention. When he took repossession of his office he found that one of his demands was for a more official Disciplinary Committee to be called the Progress Committee. Unfortunately he had then advertised for someone to run it and the appointment made under Erfert's own unique method of interviewing, had produced Matthew Brown, a man whose whole career had hitherto been spent in sending cut-off notices to the defaulting customers of the Electricity Board and whose blind devotion to this, the only trade he knew, resulted in the annual mad scramble for reassurance. His limited intellectual ability prevented him from being able to scale down his activities from that of the whole North West Region to that of a medium sized College of Education. The Electricity Board, it seemed, found it cheaper to do things on a grand scale. Thus it printed at one and the same time, bills, reminders, and cut-off notices, regardless of whether most of the reminders and cut-off notices were ever used. What might have appeared to be a rather wasteful system to anyone else was perfectly natural to Matthew Smith and, truth to tell, once understood became acceptable to the students too.

A chap called Martin Lockett explained it to Dave as the 3R's.

"The 3Rs are a sort of currency. They are Brown's Remonstrations, Rebukes and Reprimands; rather like Bills, Reminders and Cut-Off Notices. He prints them by the thousand, each on its own coloured paper, and sends them out to everyone so that no one can claim he never received one."

"And do you just bin them then?" asked the incredulous Dave.

"No, we put them to our own purposes. We use them mainly as a sort of currency in the card schools but we also have little competitions in which we out-do each other in replying to them. Our 3Rs are Replies, Rejections and Rebuttals. Some barrack- room lawyers get as far as demanding a Re-appraisal which is quite a prize."

"Why do you put up with such nonsense?"

"Oh, Matthew Brown is harmless enough. In his own eyes he is the keystone of the moral fibre of the next generation of teachers and ultimately the world. He churns out his bumph, puts in for more clerks to manage it and more space to store it and it all looks good on the peculiar indices of activity that the government apparently uses to assess efficiency these days. They allocate more money to pay for it and everyone is happy especially the suppliers of paper. Sometimes this place is so awash with bits of paper sent to all the wrong people that the college resembles Germany at the height of its hyper-inflation."

"I don't think I will put up with that for too long," said Dave.

"Now, look here Dave," warned his new friend. " I should wait a bit before getting all sanctimonious. You are new here and you have got a lot to learn. The first thing to learn is to play by the rules and not spoil anything for the rest of us."

Dave had a further surprise later when he discovered that the antics of Matthew Brown were casting further credit upon Dr Erfert. He wrote articles about his new system involving a Progress Committee rather than a Disciplinary Committee and motivation rather than sanctions. Discipline had, by a process of osmosis, become part of the Pastoral Care system. A carefully structured set of early warning signals were given and followed up with academic counselling. Students were referred to as 'consumers' rather than as passive recipients of the dry husks of learning' as they might be in other places. Each student shouldered the ultimate responsibility for his and her own progress and each personal tutor was an expert in Transactional Analysis. All this took off in a big way.

Lecturers in Australia wrote to him in admiring terms about his radical new approach to Immediate Diagnostic Monitoring Procedures. HMI's insisted that the College become a Centre of Excellence and put on In-Service courses so that the brilliant new approach could spread. Funded by the D.E.S., encouraged by its Inspectors, and its places filled by Local Authority secondees, the course was a sure-fire winner. Serving teachers, seconded by their authorities, were instantly recognisable on the campus by their mature years, complete suits, and the glazed look in the eyes which came from too much contact with Matthew

Brown. They were not going to denounce the system. They were caught in the same educational trap as everyone else. They had been sent by their bosses to get a qualification in the new and exciting venture. They dare not go back and denounce it to be the load of old rubbish that it undoubtedly was because such an opinion would reflect upon the employers who sent them, the Local Authorities who paid for them, and the Inspectors who set the whole thing up in the first place. It must be the serving teacher that was at fault because none of these august persons could be. The teacher's ability was the first thing that would be called in question and then his attitude and willingness to profit from it. The teachers were only human; they enjoyed a year out of the classroom, they wanted a qualification to further their careers, they were naturally deferential to their tutors and afforded them a professional courtesy. So they would not be devaluing the credibility of the diploma that they would be flourishing for the rest of their working lives. Whilst they might not be declaring lead to be pure gold, they would at the very least remain silent.

So Erfert continued to go from strength to strength. At the golf course and among social, rather then academic company he was brilliant because it was inconceivable that one so unintelligible could be anything else. In the academic world he had a following of fellow eccentrics, some of them in high places. At college his worst eccentricities were either covered up by saner colleagues or rebounded to his credit against all the odds. Those who felt most like rebelling against him either had a lot to lose or were of insufficient stature to make any denunciation stick. Dave was beginning to appreciate that the rules of this game were more complicated than he had realised.

Dave recognised that he had no standing even in the college nor had he much evidence or backing. He decided to play a waiting game. He could build up a dossier of evidence which would eventually convince someone someday and he would build up some credibility for himself among the students to avoid being a voice that cried in the wilderness. He might get more credibility and be in a position to collect more evidence if he sought union office or a place on the various committees or became well known at sport. Unfortunately, Dave, who was the very model of common-sense at the D.E.S, the proverbial one-eyed man in the Kingdom of the Blind, lacked a bit of common sense in all these matters. He had no real conception of the problems that he was causing himself. Getting on to the football team was no problem. He did that on the strength of having once played for Barnsley reserves. He became captain because on stripping off he proved to be the only one of the eleven who looked anything like a footballer. As he struggled to pull on his college shirt of black and red horizontal bands his colleagues beheld with admiration his barrel chest and muscular legs. He was of middle height, with no neck to speak of, and he was built on the lines of a they-shall-not-pass-the-middle-of-the-field medium tank. He had a strong constitution and a body capable of supporting the hard work that a better brain would not have asked it to do. His physical qualities matched his mental equipment in that his brains, like his muscles were just that little bit too thick. His play resembled his written work and his ideas, energetic but unimaginative, well intentioned but uninventive. He was an uncomplicated person who tackled things head on when a more subtle approach might have paid greater dividends. He was really best described as commonsense minus one. At the D.E.S, that put him ahead of most of his contemporaries but in the outside world he was just ordinary. A good deal of his character was explicable in terms of his rather possessive mother who was a great one for sticking up for her rights. She thought nothing of holding up a large queue in the supermarket whilst she insisted on having each and every item in her basket checked and re-checked. As a boy his worst moments had been when he had to accompany her on shopping trips which culminated in hostile crowds first of all shuffling and then muttering and then hurling abuse at his mother. But she, undeterred, insisted on her rights. "Pay the woman and let's get out of here while it is still daylight", they would shout. Then they would offer to pay the bill themselves if only she would move. The store manager had been known to contribute to their whip-rounds in order to get her off the premises. Like his mother, Dave was not the least bit belligerent; he just wanted his rights and he wanted to stand up for honesty and integrity when he found it impugned. Not everyone can recognise such endeavours. His way of captaining the team did not endear him to its members for instance. For him training meant running them round the edge of the pitch until they were tired, running them round again until they were dog-tired and finally running them round again until they begged for sweet release. "If it does not hurt, it does not work," he was fond of saying. He then expected them to retire straight to bed, as he did. He himself also retired to the arms of his beloved C.B. radio and to conversations under his nom de l'air "Caveman" with equally exciting people known as "Vampira" and " Dr Death".

The rest of the team had more realistic aspirations. Morale was not high when, after three weeks, the team had lost three games in a row and Dave's remedy was to run round the pitch a few more times. There was much muttering in the dressing room after one of these sessions when in walked the Principal. "Good afternoon, gentlemen," he said, smiling brightly. "I had a telephone message for Mr

Smith so I thought that I would just drop in and wish you luck for next Saturday. I understand that things have not being going your way lately. Is there anything that I can do to help?"

"Not unless you can tell us how to get a few goals," growled Dave, not averse to locking antlers with the Principal for the first time.

"Of course," came the reply from the ever obliging Erfert. "What kind of goals would you like me to explain? Ultimate, Proximate, or Mediate Goals?"

"Football goals for preference," snapped Dave, irritably.

"Much the same thing," said the Principal, happily unaware that he was being got at. "Goals in football, goals in Education, goals in life, they are all much the same you know. They are all helpful in guiding our activities in the matter of conflict resolution and they are all things that are best achieved by concerted rather than by individual effort."

"Tell that to our goalkeeper," replied Dave sourly. But such tones were lost on the happy Erfert. Dave was beginning to suspect that here was an opportunity to put one over, if not actually show up, Dr Erfert so he added in a more conciliatory tone, "but we are always ready to learn, aren't we lads?" He noted that some of the new students were nodding vigorously in the hope of escaping some of his gruelling training sessions, but several of the older hands were shaking their heads in a frantic effort to warn him off provoking yet another of Erfert's helpful ventures.

"Great," said Erfert. "I will see you all in the gym in five minutes and I will explain to you how a study of the theoretical basis can be a help to you in your efforts to overcome some of the basic problems of motivation and psycho-motor skill application."

In next to no time they were all sitting in the gym facing a blackboard, a projector screen and a shiny green board on which were placed twenty two magnetic men whilst Erfert addressed them like an academic football coach. Not for him the tracksuit and cigar. It was part of his impressive image that he was always immaculately dressed in well cut dark suits. He wore gold rimmed spectacles which made him look like a musician or a surgeon and he spoke with great confidence and with great fluency.

"Well now," he began. "As I see it you are expected to be individuals and team members at one and the same time n'est-ce-pas? You are expected to assume certain positions on the field and with those positions go some spatio-temporal areas of influence in order for you to make an effective contribution to the ritualised conflict situation in which you find yourselves. As individuals you may or not be suited to the roles assigned to you and you may or may not transmit something of your skill or your tensions to the corporate entity which, for want of a more precise word, we might call the 'team'. This in turn may generate and foster those real but intangible relationships generally known as 'team spirit' which in turn has a correlation with the scoring of goals. It is a moot point whether anyone can be expected to play a meaningful part in this process if the roles themselves have not been fully and formally defined and circumscribed. In other words, aspirational goals have to be first drawn up in a taxonomy of global objectives such as ultimate goals, proximate goals, mediate goals, exertional goals and so on. If we could get common assent on these things team selection was be relatively simple.

"We would know what would be expected of a number ten and we would know what retraining a number nine would need in order to fit in with a number ten or to replace him in the event of an injury. The rest is merely a matter of defining some behavioural objectives, clarifying the necessary and specific psycho-motor skills and establishing satisfactory lines of communication both on and off the pitch so that inter-group and intra-group and inter-personal relationships are fostered most efficiently in the conflict situation."

Dave was pleased that Erfert seemed to be making a fool of himself. He could sit back and just let it happen. When he looked round however, that was not quite the effect that Erfert was having on the assembled team. Some of those who had nodded before were now shaking their heads in disbelief but, more ominously, some of those who had shaken their heads in a vain warning were now nodding them gravely in an 'I told you so' manner.

"Adequate group functioning naturally implies the development of individual sensitivity, the recognition that one has to perform ego-orientated roles, and the management of interpersonal relations to maximise group effort. Conflict resolution begins at home, you might say."

"And just how does all this help us to win matches?" said Dave. The irony was lost on Erfert however.

"Well I think that all that running round the track is probably the wrong way to set about it," mused Erfert. He did not know it but he had now gained a good deal of interest from those who were looking for some sort of escape from Dave's brutal training regime. Even Dave could see the danger signals but before he could head off disaster one of the quicker witted students beat him to it.

"Do you think that you could explain some of this theoretical basis to us in our training sessions?" he asked innocently.

"I should be delighted to," replied Erfert who was always willing to oblige those seeking enlightenment. "It should not take more than ten or twelve lectures."

"Only ten or twelve?" asked Dave sarcastically. But again he was wasting his tone on the impervious Erfert.

"Yes, you may be right. Perhaps we need about fifteen. Shall we start tomorrow after tea? Good, see you then. Good night now." As he reached the door he suddenly turned round and remembered why he had come in the first place. "Oh, by the way Mr Smith, I completely forgot to give you a message from your mother. She says be sure to wear your woolly vest in this weather."

Dave's humiliation was complete but as yet unfinished. Erfert duly produced his course of lectures that got the team off any strenuous exercise and also informed them about the circulation of the blood of full-backs, the conservation of energy of goalkeepers and the psychological foundations of group behaviour. Instead of driving them up the wall he was saving the students from being driven up a different wall.

It also developed into something else which extended his reputation. It soon dawned on them that anyone could join the football team that did no real training at all. Girls did, disabled students did, near geriatrics did especially when he started working out new deep tactics on the computer screen. Then he started working out counter measures to his own tactics on the same computer. Then the students started working out counter-counter measures. Soon they were all playing 'real' games in deadly earnest but without the bother of getting changed or going out on to the pitch. They had evolved a new kind of sport which involved no exertion, no sweat, no showers and no bullying from Dave. A computer league was formed and this was dominated by St.Brendan's so a reputation was established.

Erfert wrote articles about simulation and gaming techniques in non aggressive conflict situations. An awful lot of people, apart from Dave, were happy. He however had lost face, although he had emerged from the episode a wiser young man. It did not lessen his determination to do something about Erfert though.

Chapter 6

Dave had learned several things at St. Brendan's. You did not tangle with Erfert unless you were ready and you needed a sense of humour if you were to survive the jibes of your friends. He had also to come to terms with the mounting piles of underclothes and other woollens which his mother sent him with every post. He consoled himself with the idea that at least she had probably not paid for them. No doubt they were the gifts of countless, anonymous, irate queues in several different supermarkets. Their generosity not only kept him warm in the winter months but also provided him with a small income on the side as he passed on their good-will gifts to his friends. They in turn nicknamed him 'Thermawear' which was a name he considered using on his C.B. rig, but he was never quite sure to whom he was talking on the rig so he decided to stick to his old name of 'Caveman'. The range of the C.B. was about five miles but any signal from close at hand tended to blot out more distant callers. So it was that the strongest signals, coming from people with handles such as 'Count Dracula', 'Batman' and 'Robin', might even be from fellow inmates of the college. One had to be careful. One particularly intriguing caller was the soft, seductive 'Delilah' who was obviously man-mad but afraid to say so.

The signal was very strong and probably emanated from close at hand. There was something familiar about the voice but he could not place it. Maybe it was distorted by the ether if not by the owner. He was on Channel Nineteen one night talking to a lorry driver who was delivering a consignment of boiled eggs to a health farm in Huddersfield when he happened to look out of the window and witnessed a sight that not only aroused his curiosity but also looked promising material for his dossier on Erfert's college. He quickly signed off and proceeded to watch the interesting spectacle that was unfolding beneath him in the gathering gloom. Two shadowy and furtive figures, not young, and not immediately recognisable as members of academic staff, were tip-toeing their way round the college buildings. The first was posting objects that looked like warning notices and the second was taking them down. The second was breaking the odd window or two and running away before the first one could catch sight of the culprit. It was all very baffling but the first thing that struck Dave was that if only he could get someone from the D.E.S. to witness this bizarre behaviour they would have to believe him. He was not to know at that point that the D.E.S. was largely responsible for the trouble in the first place.

Before it invented semesterisation and modularisation the D.E.S. went through a Health and Safety phase. It would be more accurate to say that it got frightened in case the public found out that most educational establishments failed to comply with even the minimum requirements laid down by the Health and Safety at Work Act. But being the D.E.S. the above fear also coincided with the panic that compliance might cost money. However much policy was dressed up to look like decentralisation, parental power, efficiency or quality, D.E.S. policy always came down to the same basic thing; saving money. So it was that directives went out ordering all colleges to appoint a Health and Safety Officer whose job was to report on all problems of health and safety and to recommend ways of eliminating them. At the same time, another directive went out requiring colleges to appoint a Finance Officer whose job it became in practice, to reject any such proposals if they required expenditure. That was how the scene was set for the two resident crackpots observed by Dave from his bedroom window to fight each other tooth and nail over fire-extinguishers that were not filled and emergency medical kits with nothing in them and warning notices that went up and down depending upon whether the one official wanted to warn people to watch their step or the other wanted to warn them that the college was not liable in any way shape or form for anything that might happen to them on the campus.

On the face of it, both men were good choices for the positions they held. Peter de St.Andre was not only a Belgian aristocrat but a safety fanatic. Everyday he drove just five miles to work but he did so in a new car every year. A second lay in his garage in case the first would not start. He was a member of both the A.A. and the R.A.C. in case both cars would not start and one or other of the motoring organisations could not be called out. Each car was insured with two different firms in case one went bust or in case he lost his no-claims bonus. He was just the man to look after Health and Safety.

The Finance Officer was ex-Captain William Benson whose previous exploits had included financing things on the scale of the Normandy landings and the desert campaigns of World War 11. A military man to his highly polished boots he did what he was told and the D.E.S. told him that he had to make cuts. So he called upon his knowledge of wartime ration books and quotas and he imposed a rigid regime on the rest of the college staff.

He suspected everyone of the old army trick of putting in for twice as much as was actually needed so he automatically halved all estimates even when they were fully justified. Health and safety was in need of an injection of funds because it was a relatively new thing, or perhaps a relatively neglected old thing, but not everything that St.

Andre wanted was in fact justifiable. In addition to that, Benson also considered him to be 'that long-haired, little, foreign, conscientious objector' who was trying to break the bank. So he took great personal delight in refusing to sign even the most reasonable request from that quarter. The more the reasonable requests were refused the more unreasonable became the requests and the more irate became the Health and Safety man. He took some revenge by closing down whole sections of the college on health and safety grounds or insisting on the remodelling of specialist rooms on the grounds that they were unsafe. He disrupted many an afternoon with his fire-drills and regularly threatened to close down the kitchens for lack of hygiene.

All this posed a problem for Captain Benson. He knew that he could be in deep trouble if he refused to implement recommendations and someone was injured because of it but he could not bring himself to comply with the recommendations of somebody whom he suspected of having been planted behind British lines (albeit as an infant) in order to emerge as a saboteur in our hour of need. So he usually managed not to receive the requests, or else he mislaid them, or else he found fault with the wording, the address or the signature. It was all very time-consuming. Open warfare was rare; trench warfare more the normal order of the day. Sometimes St.Andre got his own back with a vengeance. During the summer holidays it was customary for the college to be hired out for conferences and courses because the D.E.S expected an entrepreneurial, business-like management of resources. This made money for the college and it also led to one or two perks for Captain Benson which he was anxious not to lose.

The Health and Safety Officer had it within his power to make life hell for Benson on these occasions without hurting any of the staff or students of St. Brendan's. He had ways of frightening guests in subtle ways such as calling in a Rento-Kill firm to fumigate the beds just before the startled guests were to retire for the night or else turning off all the water supplies so that guests were reduced to collecting jugs of the stuff from central standpipes. It was all good 1940's stuff but it failed to appeal to Captain Benson. He was reduced to booking conferences only in the weeks when he knew St.Andre was on holiday or else to bribing him by signing orders in the weeks before the conferences.

It was during one of the conferences that a guest slipped on a badly laid paving stone and fractured a wrist. The Safety Officer surprised him by urging him to sue the college for every penny he could get, to complain to the Finance Officer and to summon the Safety Officer as a willing witness to the event he had not in fact seen. The Finance Officer surprised him even more by demanding to know by what right he had been trespassing upon a piece of private college land.

"But it was a footpath. It was six feet wide and obviously laid for people to walk to dining room," he protested.

"Prove it," snarled the military man.

"I don't have to prove it," snorted the man indignantly."You prove that it isn't."

"Right," said Benson, and he promptly took out from his desk a notice on which was printed; 'Keep Off. Trespassers will be prosecuted'.

He then took the notice and the bewildered guest to the spot where the accident had happened and plonked the notice right in the middle of the path. "There, that plainly shows that you have no right to walk there. If you do so you have only yourself to blame. I think you will find that we are in the clear." With that he photographed the man standing next to the notice and marched off in triumph.

St. Andre vowed a terrible revenge. The form this took was a visit from the Gas Board after he persuaded the irate guest that they both could smell gas in the room of the Finance Officer. His own specialist opinion was taken seriously by the Gas Board inspectors who promptly tipped Benson out of his room and ripped up his composition floor so that he could not return. It took Benson two days to remove all his files to another room and it took St. Andre just three days to have him tipped out of it by his faithful band of gas workers. Thus he discovered a cheap and cheerful way of exacting a sweet revenge. And he still had in reserve the Water Board, the Electricity Board and the Public Health Officers of the Local Authority. They would all turn out for nothing on the word of someone with a high-sounding title. Moreover they could be targeted in a selective manner towards his arch enemy and not towards innocent students or guests of the college.

In desperation the Finance Officer took himself and his clerk to a caravan parked outside the main administration block only to discover that someone had reported it to the police for having some dangerous metal strips protruding from the side-embellishments. It was also left unlit at night and constituted a hazard to other vehicles, the temperature inside did not conform to those laid down for offices and there was insufficient cubic capacity to maintain the presence of both the Finance Officer and his clerk at the same time. The feud would have ended in bloodshed had not Nemesis intervened. As the Safety Officer was directing the Gas Board workmen to a possible gas leak under the caravan he suddenly disappeared into the exploratory hole which they had just dug nearby. Having no-one to sue for his injury, he accepted the Finance Officer's generous offer that he should take six month's paid leave of absence. Dave had witnessed his return and the start of a new round of guerrilla warfare.

Chapter 7

After all his setbacks Dave was looking forward to mid-term and to a much needed break. It would also give him a chance to chat to his father who was a sensible man, willing to give advice but not to interfere. His father shared his mother's sense of right and wrong but not her obstinacy in pursuing just causes. He also had a better sense of humour than either his wife or his son. He particularly enjoyed Dave's mournful stories of his first college experiences and found Frederick Toser's History lecturing style the most amusing of all. Frederick Toser was renowned in the History Department (now renamed Chronological Data Retrieval Services) because of his psychological approach to the interpretation of historical figures and because of his tendency to recount historical situations by roundly ticking off Napoleon or Henry V111 for not doing what Toser thought in retrospect that they ought to have attempted. He also gave them a free retrospective psycho-analysis. To him, Bismarck was a big, coarse Junker on the outside, like his father, but on the inside he was his soft, delicate, intelligent mother. His role in History and the mistakes he made were all put down to the one Bismarck masquerading as the other. Toser regarded himself as being in a position to tell Bismarck and anyone else who would listen where History had gone wrong and what ought to have happened if only they could have listened to him.

"That reminds me of the old Irish story," chuckled his father.

"There was this old Irish woman whose husband had died and she was telling the neighbour that the post-mortem had told them the cause of death. She said that if only he had had the post-mortem before he died, they could have saved him." He then went on to say, "seriously though, you are wasting your time, you know. You will never win."

"Why not?" demanded Dave.

"Well, for a start you can't hold Erfert responsible for the antics of any individual members of staff even though he may be responsible. Toser is presumably a qualified historian, you are not. He is probably a qualified teacher, you are not. You don't find members of the public getting far if they criticise doctors or dentists do you?"

"That's different," grumbled Dave.

"What's different about it? You and I both know that there are incompetents in every profession; there are also some who are competent but should never be let near students or children. But you need to be a saner, senior, competent, person yourself, before anyone will listen to you."

"I might be able to get the D.E.S. to do something about it."

"You really think so? What makes you think that they don't know all about it ? Or would do something about it? I deal with the D.E.S every day of the week and you will find more idiots per square foot of Elizabeth house than almost anywhere else. The difference is that they make the rules and so they are always right. Do you know who had a hand in appointing Erfert to St. Brendan's in the first place? None other than Sir Kenneth Michael, your former Secretary of State for Education and Science."

That clinched it for Dave. Sir Kenneth Michael was recognised as being something of an embarrassment even by the D.E.S. His mind went back to the story of how Sir Kenneth had insisted on appointing a personal adviser straight from Winchester and Trinity who had promptly announced to the press that he was to give objective advice in that he had never been in a state school in his life, and when he did visit a few, like a colonial administrator, he embarrassed everyone by asking poor children if they did not have higher aspirations in life than being hewers of wood and drawers of water. The absurdity of a system administered by people who had no knowledge of it, no sympathy with it, no vested interest in it had never really struck him when he had been immersed in the administrative details of running this colonial empire.

"What am I supposed to do then?" Dave wanted to know.

"Forget the D.E.S. You will get no help from them. They will be glad to see the back of you and your next career move will already be on file, labelled 'Oblivion'. If I were you I would go through with the course. Get yourself professionally qualified and have something to fall back on when they give you the push. You will also be in a better position to get people to listen to you if you still want to get at Erfert. If all else fails you can always teach. Who knows, you may even like it."

"I doubt it," shuddered Dave, appalled at the prospect.

"See what I mean about the D.E.S.? I bet you did not say that when you were helping to run the system. My advice is to sit back, relax, get yourself a nice girl, a

69

teaching qualification ,and," he added with a twinkle in his eye, " be sure to wear your woollies."

Dave thought about this advice all the way back to college. He was still thinking about it when he passed through the main gate only to be hailed by the porter who said he had a message for him from the Principal. The message was a curious one. "Dear Mr Smith," it began, "I am sorry to bother you but I have tried without success to contact one of our students, Arthur Pitts. As I understand that he is a friend of yours and a member of your football team, I wonder if I could ask you to contact him for me? Alternatively you might be able to provide me with some of the information that I require. Has he been baptised for instance? Have you been baptised yourself, by the way? Never mind that. It is just Arthur Pitts I am interested in at the moment. I am also pleased to tell you that you have been elected to be the students' representative on the College Academic Board. Congratulations."

Chapter 8

On arriving back at college after his thirty fifth baptism the Principal was confronted with several items of correspondence. Most men in his position would have found that something of a bore but he revelled in it. His particular forte was answering daft questions with equally silly replies - not that he or any of the recipients would have recognised them to be such. This was partly due to the fact that the D.E.S. had different departments churning out masses of contradictory requests, instructions and advice. Thus, in the same post, they had sent him two contradictory requests. The one asked what he was doing to make the small group of postgraduate students feel more like a homogeneous group, a cohesive unit, a recognisable group with an identity of its own; the other was demanding to know what he was doing to integrate the small group of postgraduate students into the life of the college and, in particular, what steps was he taking to avoid their natural pretensions to become a small elitist group. Erfert managed to answer both questions satisfactorily. In answer to the first letter he replied that he had allocated these students a special room where they could feel at home and establish a group identity; special funds had been set aside to help them do this; special lapel badges would help them to recognise each other. To the second letter he reported that he had decided to disperse these students throughout the college and had taken away such things as a special common room and special monies which might make them something of a privileged class. He was not doing this out of a cynical disregard for the truth but because he had a kind of schizophrenic amnesia. At the time of writing he sincerely believed in what he was doing. The first letter stirred him to action but so did the second sometime later and when he discovered that these students were being treated like an elite he put the matter right at once.

At the D.E.S. it did not matter anyway because the two letters landed on two different desks in two different departments whilst a third department was considering the possibility of taking the postgraduate course out of colleges altogether and putting it in the hands of teachers in schools, much to the chagrin of the fourth department which was announcing that teachers in schools were badly trained and not fit to teach pupils let alone future teachers.

Once he had dealt with the correspondence he looked up the directory that contained the names of all the local churches and their clergymen within a thirty mile radius of the college in order to settle upon a suitable place in which to have his thirty-sixth baptism. He had long since run out of local clergymen to perform this function. His problem in religion was not unlike his problem in education. In thinking too much he was capable of constructing the most fantastic schemes out of basically reasonable propositions. He believed, along with millions of others that 'Unless a man be born again of water and the Holy Ghost he shall not enter into the Kingdom of Heaven' but his further reading had led him to believe that only one hundred and forty four thousand souls would be allowed entry into Paradise. His mathematical bent together with his historical knowledge and his famous problem-solving technique told him that the majority must have taken up their places before now so that a person coming late upon the scene as in the twentieth century would have to make very sure of his entrance qualifications as soon as possible.

Infancy was as good a start as any but he started thinking deeply about Baptism being a sort of eleven plus entrance qualification and the possibility of its being validly or invalidly administered by worthy and unworthy priests. Obviously not any Tom, Dick or Harry would do and he had no idea of the character of the man who had first carried out his own infant Baptism. So he looked around in adult life for some minister or priest whose own personal sanctity would make it reasonable to suppose that the sacrament had in fact been validly administered. He carefully built up secret dossiers on all the local clergy before he approached them to baptise him but he found none of them beyond reproach. Most of them had performed the ceremony for him as requested and some of the more perceptive had thrown in an exorcism as well without his knowledge but he was still not satisfied. He watched the ceremony like a hawk to make sure that everything was done in the approved manner and he continued to investigate the personal lives of the clergy to make sure that the efficacy of the sacrament was not invalidated by any personal failings on their part. After thirty five attempts he had still not found a perfect ceremony or a worthy priest or virtuous vicar and the odds against his doing so were rising every year. Once the vicar knew of his interest in his performance and his integrity he tended to go to pieces and make lots of mistakes. Erfert got more and more worried the more he found defective ceremonies. Not just on his own account but for all the millions of people who mistakenly believed themselves to be validly baptised by such incompetents. So he went on his merry way through an ever widening circle around the college, the scourge of local and not so local clergymen. Some refused to baptise him and he had to resort to false names and disguises.

That also worried him in case he himself was invalidating the sacrament. But the ex-Jesuit and father of six whom he had appointed as Head of R.E. came to his aid by supplying a doctrine of mental reservation that appealed to his vein of casuistry. Michael O'Hara had reminded him of the various dodges that the Jesuits had used in the days of the Elizabethan persecution of priests. So, if a vicar asked if he had been baptised before, Erfert would reply; "Would to God that I had been properly baptised" or he might say, "It is my dearest wish to be baptised properly." If he were asked his name he would say, "I come before you as a sinner, one Harry Jones." These stratagems had worked for some time but now he was running out of vicars. To some of advanced years or defective vision he had been twice or thrice but there was always some doubt about the validity of sacraments administered by such persons in any case. To others he dare not show his face. Michael O'Hara was able to put his mind at rest about being baptised in other people's names. It was either a valid ceremony or it was not, he pointed out. If it was not, then the false name did not matter. If it was a valid ceremony then two things could happen. Either it was valid for him as the recipient regardless of name, or the name really mattered. In the first case he benefited; in the second case someone else did. Either way he was doing a bit of good in the world. Thereafter it pleased him to be an anonymous proxy for lots of his agnostic and atheistic friends and students. His only regret was that Michael O'Hara himself seemed to be disqualified from performing a valid ceremony by virtue of a technicality in the shape of his wife and six children. He also had a few doubts about some of the subtleties suggested by O'Hara to solve his own problems and this prompted one of his wiser sayings; "They are clever people, all right, these Jesuits, but I wouldn't let my daughter marry one."

His motive in all this was an inner craving for certainty. He was not a pious man but he was always kind and considerate to others. Except that is on the occasion when a fit of religious mania compelled him to tell the strict truth to people in circumstances when the truth was best left on the back burner. The problem would not have been so bad if it had not coincided with the onset of one of his Educational Management theories known later as the theory of Constructive Conflict. The fact that he was telling people the truth was enough to generate plenty of conflict without any backing from the theory but the combination led to a situation where many people were not on speaking terms for many a long day. Mrs. Sudden was the first recipient of his new style of leadership. She was a formidable lady in her own right but she was completely taken aback when her polite "Good Morning" was met with a scornful comment that that was a banal remark that everyone was making without regard to the actual state of the weather.

"I am sorry I spoke," said she in a huff.

"Never mind," countered Erfert. "We cannot all rise above the obvious cliché and it must be difficult to think in that hat."

"What is wrong with my hat?" she demanded to know.

"It is pretty hideous. Do you wear it to take the attention off the dress?"

He was actually saying all this in his usual smiling way but trying out his theory of constructive conflict by telling the truth but Mrs. Sudden did not see it that way. She had not the eccentricity of some of his zanier appointees to take this sort of thing in her stride or tell him to ".... Off " as did the monosyllabic Art man.

Mr Scott's "I think that it is going to be fine for the Test Match today." was greeted with the statement that Erfert could not care less. And in truth he could *not* care less. He was not trying to hurt anyone. He was just waiting for something constructive to arise out of the conflict. Everyone he met he insulted in a most courteous manner often by simply telling the literal truth but sometimes by deliberately goading them. On occasion it had surprising results as when he phoned the Finance Officer.

"Look Bill," he said in the friendliest of tones, "just put Miss Jones down for a moment and tell me the state of the Field-Work account. Use the real book and not the one you show to the auditors." There was a strangled gasp at the other end of the line.

"Yes sir, of course, sir," said the startled Captain Benson who hastily put down his accounts clerk and dutifully supplied the Principal with accurate information from a secret ledger marked 'Pension Fund'. Whether the Principal knew something, whether he was repeating hearsay, or whether his theory of constructive conflict had prompted him to say something provocative is not possible to ascertain, but the college accounts certainly took on a cleaner and fresher look from that day forward.

Shortly after that episode the Head of Economics went into the Principal's office to ask about some extra funds for a projected field trip. He was first of all delighted to be told that the Finance Officer had enough funds to pay out and then dismayed to be informed that some of the staff considered Economics to be an immature pseudo-science which needed all the money it could get if it were ever to achieve respectability. He crawled out of the office vowing revenge on whichever colleagues had given that opinion to the Principal. Storming into the staff room he found two irate scientists wrestling about the floor as one tried to destroy and the other defend, Mrs Sudden's hideous hat, all to the accompaniment of her hysterical background wails.

Soon the Academic Board met to discuss this bizarre situation and the Principal was happy to explain the value of Constructive Conflict to the staff gathered around the impressive old oak table. His opening was not auspicious because of the difficulty in getting order and then of getting through to the deafest member of staff sitting furthest away from him.

"Would you speak up at the front please?" said the deaf man in a murmur.

"Would you speak up at the back please?" said Erfert who could not make out what he had said.

"Shut up," said the monosyllabic Art man, and that seemed to settle it.

When he finally did explain why he at least had been so rude the Principal surpassed even his heights of semi-plausible nonsense.

"I have developed the theory of Constructive Conflict because, like other people, we have all become a bit too complacent. We all get on too well with each other. What we need is a shake-up, a re-appraisal of our role-playing procedures. The best way to do that is to have a grass-roots reconsideration of our conventional politeness and our rituals so that we can reveal the inner dynamism of our goal-based assumptions. We can have a meaningful dialogue with each other but above all with ourselves, and emerge from the experience in a new and purer form. I like to think of it as a purgatorial re-alignment."

"Any questions?" he asked.

"Yes," said Mrs Sudden. "Can I take it then that you really did not dislike my hat and that you were only trying to provoke me into being whatever it was that you just described?"

"No, not really," said Erfert, the religious nut, "It would not be honest of me to say that I like your hat. In fact I think that your hat is something of a disaster and will be all the better for the beating up that I understand it received in the staff room the other day."

Her screams could be heard a mile away and the Board broke up in disorder. A vote of no confidence in the chairman could hardly be heard because of the hysterical cries of Mrs Sudden and the noise of his loony supporters singing "We shall overcome" at the tops of their voices. Erfert took it all as evidence that his new theory was a brilliant success. In one sense it was a brilliant success because, after it, the college benefited from the same desire for peace which exhausted European nations have exhibited after each world war.

Dave, the student representative on the Academic Board made notes but even he was under no illusion that anyone would believe him.

Chapter 9

Dave was sitting in the Lecture given by one of the resident weirdo's in Educational Psychology but he was paying more attention to a rather nice looking, dark haired girl who, like most of the other girls, was busy taking down notes on the nonsense that was being delivered. The lecture was on rats and mice and anything else in the animal kingdom except young children. After all the dogs salivated to stimuli, the lecturer somehow linked it with unidirectional thinking and ego-centricity in the pre-operational stage of reasoning but Dave just groaned and read yet again the messages scratched into the desk lid to the effect that Liverpool supporters were of doubtful parentage. The girl gave him a sympathetic look but continued to take down great spoonfuls of the jollop.

"Fancy a coffee?" He mouthed at her.

"OK," she whispered back as the lecturer finished on the skills of Analysis, Synthesis, and Extrapolation that could be found even in so called simple psycho-motor activities.

"What's the matter? Are you not happy here?" she asked when they settled down to a coffee in the snack bar.

"I wasn't happy when I came and I am a damn sight less happy now," he confessed, without revealing anything about his real motives for coming or staying.

"But what is wrong with it?" she persisted.

"It's like Alice in Wonderland," he replied, "and that last lunatic is the Mad Hatter. No he isn't, Erfert is."

"Well he is a bit strange, I grant you but he is really a very nice man and he is very highly thought of. I am baby-sitting for him tonight"

"He is a lunatic but I don't suppose anyone will agree with me," grumbled Dave, but he didn't pursue it because his mind was already working out how he could get baby-sitting with her that night. Here again the gods were against him for the "baby" in question was Erfert's obnoxious son, Brian. In the end he decided that the girl was worth the risk.

Just at that moment Brian was the subject of a conversation between Dr.Erfert and his long-suffering wife.

"Do you think that Brian will be good for the baby-sitter tonight?" she asked anxiously. "Perhaps it would be better to stay in."

"Nonsense, my dear," replied Erfert. "It would be foolish to give up now just when I am getting somewhere with the Chief Education Officer. And it is all for Brian's good you know."

His wife groaned for he was referring to a meeting that night with the local Chief Education Officer to discuss Erfert's plan to have his son educated in what was then called an Approved School. Understandably, the C.E.O. had at first treated it as a joke derived from the great man's sense of humour but the doctor was as persistent as he was serious. He did not see why his son should miss out on what some people regarded as the best education in the country. It certainly was, in terms of the cash poured into it, the advantageous staffing ratios that it enjoyed, the lavishly equipped specialist rooms and the strong moral tone that pervaded its disciplined approach. Such schools had a more advantageous capitation allowance than either Eton or Harrow but, like Eton and Harrow, the benefits were confined to a privileged few.

His wife had, as always, tried to put him off his hair-brained scheme. "I think that Brian is happy where he is, dear," she ventured. "Could he not stay a little longer, at least until he gets to know the girls better?" She was referring to the all-girls school which the little blighter attended after his father had fought tooth and nail to get him admitted on the principle of equal opportunities.

"I am afraid that I have lost confidence in that place," replied Erfert. "I wish that I had known that they still believed in class teaching when I sent him there." He loved his son but his well meaning attempts to have him educated according to the best educational practices had produced a little monster. From birth to the age of five he had been reared according to the "Natural" tradition of Rousseau. Until the age of seven he had come under the influence of the Jesuits on the assumption that the famous quotation of Ignatius Loyola was a valid maxim.

Before reaching his present unenviable stage he had been subjected to the theories of Pestalozzi, Herbart, Froebel, Bell, Lancaster and Montessori. It was only when Mrs Erfert had caught her husband reading a prospectus for the training of Hitler Youth that she had threatened to have the boy kidnapped by gypsies rather than have him go through another change of direction. Although quite interested in the gypsy suggestion, Erfert had settled upon the all-girls school run by nuns. It seemed a sensible compromise between the Jesuits and the Hitler Youth. Brought up in this fashion, by a famous educationist father, it is not surprising that the boy Brian was a little swine, detested by all for his smirking countenance, his nasty habits, his bad manners and his incredible combination of esoteric knowledge and plain, unvarnished ignorance. He had never really got over the fact that there were at least three learned articles about his early childhood in which his every move had been recorded and interpreted to that level of sophistication which was little short of insanity. During the school holidays his father had often taken him to commune with nature on the Yorkshire moors in order to teach him self reliance and the ability to think for himself. Erfert judged this to be satisfactorily completed when he had been told by his son to "stuff" his lessons. If the truth were known an Approved School was just the place for this young man but with Erfert it was a matter of principle unconnected with his son's obvious qualifications.

So it was that Jane had been asked to baby-sit whilst he and his wife went to persuade the Chief Education Officer to agree with his request. The latter had tried ignoring it, denying receiving it, and positively refusing it and now he had finally agreed to give Erfert a personal hearing in his own home because of the great man's reputation. Mrs Erfert had a worried look on her face as she opened the door to the young couple, for Dave had managed to get himself invited too. She appeared to him to be a trifle over-fussy about the arrangements.

"Now here is the telephone number where we can be contacted," she said, "and on the pad near the telephone are the numbers of the emergency services such as the Fire Brigade and the Gas Board. I am afraid that they won't answer 999 calls from this house any more but if you ring the police directly you can usually get them to come out. I am sure you won't need them but I thought that I would leave them just in case." There was something about her anxious tone that started a 999 bell ringing in Dave's head especially when she went on to assure Jane that; "I am so glad that you brought Dave along, I know that you will be all right with a strong young man to protect you."

"It can't be that bad," thought Dave, but it was.

The place was booby-trapped. The cushions let out rude noises when depressed. Foul smells emanated from innumerable stink bombs. The television set, radio and CD player were all blaring away and the boy was constantly hungry or thirsty. Dave must have made twenty or thirty trips to the kitchen to keep him supplied and on several occasions had to make a hasty return in order to prevent Jane being indecently assaulted. Then, in strict contravention of all that he had learned in Psychology, Dave belted him with a large cane which he removed from a plant pot for the purpose. This reduced Brian to outraged tears and dire threats that Dave would not only be out on his ear next morning but also that his career was over and he would be lucky not to be dragged through the courts by the parents on their return.

They in the meantime were being entertained by the C.E.O. He was a man who had come up the hard way. At least he had always found it hard to explain to people that he was the son-in-law of the Chairman of the Education Committee. But he was no mug although no match for his visitor.

"You are very welcome," he assured them. "It is a great pleasure to meet you again. I have to warn you, however, that I do not see how I can accede to your rather unusual request."

"Why not?" asked Erfert, innocently.

"Well it is just not normal for ordinary boys to go to an Approved School. Surely you are aware of that ?"

"I am aware that the policy of the government and of the Education Committee here is to do away with privilege, segregation and selection. Is that not so?"

"Well of course it is," he spluttered, "but that is for ordinary pupils in ordinary schools. You do not want your son mixing with riff-raff do you?"

"Are they not in ordinary schools before they go to Approved School?" asked Erfert.

The C.E.O. nodded.

"And do they not return to ordinary schools as ordinary pupils after their spell in the Approved School?"

The C.E.O. again nodded assent.

"So they are only not ordinary pupils whilst there?"

"I suppose so."

"But are they not treated as ordinary pupils whilst there?"

"Yes, of course."

"Then what is your point?"

The C.E.O couldn't quite remember what his point was so Erfert continued. "Is it not a fact that the Local Authority has to consider the wishes of parents when allocating children to school?"

"Yes"

"Even if that means a school outside the borough?"

"Yes."

"Or a Church school?"

"Yes."

"Why draw the line at an Approved School then?"

"Because no-one wants to send their children to an Approved School."

"How do you know that? Is one listed on the options list?"

"No."

"If it is not an option how can they choose it? You did not know for instance that I myself wanted to avail of this option did you?"

"Not until I received your letter."

"Well as I see it, the 1988 Act as amended gives me the right to express my wishes in the matter so I want to exercise my right. Other people may do the same if only they got the chance. You do not tell people their rights and then point to the absence of letters to claim that everyone agrees with your policy. I also see it as one way in which the working classes are receiving more favourable treatment than the middle classes."

"But parents do not have an absolute right to have their wishes fulfilled. Other considerations come into it like distance and expense."

"Oh I have gone into all that," Erfert assured him. "The school I want is nearer to my house than the local secondary school; it is a denominational school and it is all-boys. I want to exercise my right to have my boy educated in a single-sex, Catholic, Approved School near my home and with a much better teacher/pupil ratio than any of the other schools in the area. I am considering asking the Secretary of State to intervene using her powers under section 68 of the 1944 Education Act."

"But boys have to be sent to an Approved School. They have to go before a court and they are sent there as a punishment."

"That does not sound very fair on the girls to me," responded Erfert. "Middle class girls could hardly be expected to qualify by that route, to be sure. But of course I deny your premise that Education is to be seen as a punishment. I am sure that if you reflect you will see that such a notion is a negation of all that the Approved School is supposed to stand for. If anything it is an institution for the improvement of boys not for their punishment and , that being so, I want my son to be improved in a school that has been specifically designed and equipped for that purpose. I am thinking of getting the court to grant me a writ of

Mandamus against the Local Authority for refusing my rights in the matter of choice of school."

He said all this very quietly and with great good nature but he had all the determination of the genuine fanatic. The C.E.O was not clever enough to cope with him but he was quick enough to spot the threat to his Authority and to his father-in law. He knew his officials would find some way round the problem and he put Erfert on hold for the evening whilst he offered them a sherry. In the event he need not have worried for the boy found his own way into the Approved school a short time later by way of the local shopping precinct and the magistrates court. His father proved to be delighted with the progress he made there and was only a little unhappy about the restricted home visiting.

On their return home Dave was naturally anxious about the consequences of his brutality but Erfert seemed to think corporal punishment worthy of debate rather than censure and his wife pulled Dave to one side and assured him that it might do Brian a bit of good. She would personally see to it that his career did not suffer for it. Dave, for his part, thought a little better of Erfert if only because a man who had won such a woman could not be all bad. It was no bad thing that Jane regarded him as something of a saviour knight either.

Chapter 10

"I give up," moaned Dave in despair.

"Whatever is the matter?"asked a concerned Jane.

"I have just been to Erfert's house to collect a book
that we left there when we were criminal-sitting and the
door was answered by a beery-looking character who swore
at me, told me that he was the Principal and that I was to
push off before I got a faceful of knuckles."

She had no answer to that one. The answer lay in a
devastating combination of one of Erfert's theories with the
dubious activities of chief spiv and specialist in P.E,
Michael Schofield. Just what aspect of P.E. that Schofield
specialised in was something of a mystery for he had never
been seen to leave the ground or even to quicken his pace
unless it were in search of a quick buck. In some circles he
would have merited the appellation 'Entrepreneur' but
basically he was a crook. He couldn't even visit the local
superstore without feeding his children before reaching the
checkout and then having the cheek to present large
numbers of cash-off coupons that he had just stripped from
the tins on the shelves. He rarely used cash, preferring his
own version of the circulation of money, paying for most
things with a Barclaycard, paying the card debt with a
Barclayloan, paying the interest on the Barclayloan by using
an Access card. Underpinning the Access card was a little

business he had built up through which he advertised and sold a pill to pregnant women which ensured that they had boy babies. If they did not have a boy baby he gave them their money back. The result was a nice little earner as nature provided him with a steady income on fifty percent of all clients.

It was only natural that the staff looked to Schofield for the organisation of various social events, and it was just as natural that he should make a packet out of doing so. He had booked typical Majorcan clog dancers with suspicious accents and even more suspicious suntans. He had booked leading dance bands who had been dogged with such ill luck as to be delayed by road conditions or dysentery. His coloured Blues Singers were strangely reluctant to wipe their dripping coloured brows and when they did they tended, like the clog dancers and the dance bands, to bear a distinct resemblance to members of his own family, particularly his boozy brother-in-law. It was not generally known that this man drank until one day he came sober and on time and his act was even more terrible than usual. But Going-Down Dinners were not the place to find sober discerning audiences anyway. This brother-in-law was at the centre of most of Schofield's ventures. He could always be spotted in the group when the P.E. man rented groups of students to unscrupulous T.V producers wanting to film student unrest or when the students wanted to hire pieces of craft work for submission to the examiners. "Odd-Job" as he was known because of his resemblance to a James Bond character, bought up a collection of genuine exhibits from leaving students and then produced them year after year for the talentless to pass off as their own work. Each one was carefully catalogued in terms of origins, date of submission and previous marks gained. As examiners were appointed for three years these ladies and gentlemen were also on file and cross matched with the artefacts.

Schofield and his relative had in fact brought order and improvement to a previous system in which desperate students had attempted to pass off such things as whitewood furniture and stripped-down, shop-bought chairs, as their own.

The one thing that Schofield could not fix was the appointment of a new Principal and when Erfert had appeared on the scene it looked as if his activities would cease forthwith. He spent long hours rehearsing what he would say to the new man if he delved into his past misconduct.

His chance came when Erfert sent for him.

"For some years now," explained Erfert before Schofield could get out his alibi, "I have been trying to overcome one of the fundamental problems of educational research, the Hawthorne Effect. As you know this is when an investigation is spoiled by the fact that the subjects know that they are the subjects of an investigation and act accordingly. If only we could devise a research experiment, here for instance, without the people concerned knowing that they were under investigation, think how much more valuable that would be."

"So you want to disguise it in some way?"

"Yes, I want someone to take my place while I conduct the investigation undetected as it were."

"Is that going to fool anybody?"

"It will if you find me a double. Can you do that?"

"Of course," said Mike with all the old confidence returning after his initial fear had worn off. "Of course, when I say a double, I do not necessarily mean someone who is identical to yourself."

He was surprised to see Erfert nodding at that.

"You see," added Mike, "we all have a self image of ourselves which is never the real person. We do not even have a real image in a mirror so we never really know what the real 'me' is. That being so we have no real means of comparing ourselves with a double, have we? Even the mirror image is only a reflected and distorted version of ourselves and we never really know how we look, or sound or appear to others either. So, in finding you a double I am not going to kid you into thinking that I am getting someone identical to you in a superficial sense. I am going to get you someone who resembles the real you as I see it." He did not add that the double would also be remarkably like his brother-in-law.

"Capital," agreed a delighted Erfert, "the double need not be identical."

They then planned the changeover when the double would be smuggled into College to take Erfert's place and Erfert would merge into the background in order to observe the rest of the College from a privileged position and penetrate the real network of relationships that might otherwise prove to be so elusive. It would be an exciting and enlightening way of discovering groups and subgroups in the formal and the informal structure and infrastructure. That was how the brother-in-law came to be running St.

Brendan's for a short while and how Dr Erfert became a temporary gardener roaming the College in the fond belief that he was incognito, to observe and to record from behind trees and hedges. The fact that the 'new' Principal had left school at fifteen and had a vocabulary that would have shamed a sailor's parrot made for even less credibility but Erfert got a good article out of it nevertheless. Engaging the brother-in-law proved to be easier than dismissing him, however, and, failing to get the compensation he demanded, he would return from time to time to continue his new profession. Most people, including Erfert learned to tolerate him but meeting him for the first time, as did Dave, was an unnerving experience.

Chapter 11

It was a tired Dave Smith who wandered through the corridors of St Brendan's in search of his lecture on Primary Mathematics to be delivered by Dr Erfert himself. He had not had much sleep after the late night before and was not thinking too clearly when he stumbled upon a five pound note lying on the floor of the lecture room just inside the doorway. He instinctively stooped to pick it up only to be startled by a huge cheer from the assembled students inside. He looked round to find the Principal winding in the cotton attached to the note and pulling the latter tantalisingly out of Dave's reach.

"That's another one," shouted the delighted academic. "That makes twenty-one I think."

At that figure he seemed to lose interest in his psychological experiment and launched into a lecture on probability and graphs. It was in fact more interesting than the average Education lecture. Normally it would consist of strict admonitions not to lecture to children by a person who knew no other trade himself. The lecturer, often not on speaking terms with his colleagues, would also insist that the teacher should have declared aims and objectives which were commonly agreed by the staff and parents alike. Tame psychologists vied with sociologists and philosophers to be primus inter pares in the so-called science of Education, each pursuing his own discipline as if it were the Queen of all Sciences.

Dave quite liked History lectures, boring though they often were. The fact that you could pick and choose from a huge quantity of material something that interested you was a source of quiet satisfaction to the average student. He was surprised to find that it was not all memory work but could require some intelligent thinking on occasion.

English was a different kettle of fish, however. There is obviously something about northerners which makes them incapable of appreciating the finer things in life, things like the ballet or poetry. Even the admission that he liked Rugby League and pigeon racing could be interpreted as inverted snobbery by those who dictated the cultural norms of the college. If anyone could interpret anything thus, it was surely his fastidious English lecturer, Miss Greta Morgan-Power.

She had first caught him out for mis-pronouncing one of the more obscure Oxford College names and then she found fault with his northern vowels which, she complained, ruined the rhythm, or the rhyme, or the metre or the meaning or the message of the poetry which she was desperately trying to get the group to enjoy.

She, on the other hand, prided herself on her inflexions, on her perfect pronunciation and on her acting ability. She also made a point of dressing up in appropriate costume for each reading. A surprising number of poems thus read required her wear a crinoline. Such a person could hardly be expected to take to a rugby-loving Yorkshireman and she soon gave it as her opinion that he would be happier studying Geography, a subject which would permit him to tramp all over the countryside in great big muddy boots. This in itself was a poetic way of describing what he was already doing to her sacred ground.

Her great forte was to detect the author's message, preferably hidden, in the piece of work before them. One of

Dave's claims to fame at the D.E.S. had been to liaise with various authors who had contributed to a book of verse that the Department intended to impose on schools as part of a National Curriculum package. In that capacity he had got to know several authors quite well. He had even had a pint or two with some of the less affected specimens. He knew well enough that some of the hidden messages that Greta Morgan-Power was finding in their work were just too ridiculous for words. He thought that inside knowledge might be useful to him and it might also help him to show-up his precious tutor. As in most other matters connected with St. Brendan's, he could not have been more wrong. Greta Morgan-Power was not the least bit interested in what the author actually thought. She insisted in telling the group at great length what the author obviously intended to write. Her method of teaching was to assemble a group of students in a small tutorial room, reading the poem in a very dramatic fashion and demanding to know what was the hidden message that lay behind the words. She could not be persuaded that there might not be a hidden message to discover so the students became adept at interpreting the poems in the way she wanted. All except Dave. He knew for a fact that one of the poems had only entered the book because he and the author had had a night on the tiles and had been written in a pub on the back of an envelope before Dave had accepted it for publication.

The Tutor struck a pose as she recited;

"If you were here where all is mild,
And I could find a baby-sitter,
I would not shirk what I must pay,
To contemplate the bitter."

Her version of the hidden message became deeper and deeper as it evolved.

"The first thing that comes to mind is that this is a plea from a married man who is seeking reconciliation with his estranged wife. He has obviously achieved a certain amount of peace and tranquillity after the initial trauma but now realises what he has lost and he is willing to do anything, to pay any price, to make it up to her. He or she is in fact the real hero or heroine of the piece, but a tragic one I fear, probably handicapped; the word 'bitter' would lead us to suspect that. Maybe it is a triangle of an estranged couple and a handicapped child that gives a special poignancy to the word 'bitter'. Of course the word 'you' in line one might lead us to an even more interesting interpretation. It might be that the lady is not his wife at all and that he is involved in an extra-marital relationship. All is 'mild' i.e.stale, in his marriage, but if only she would join him in a ménage a trois, perhaps masquerading as a baby-sitter it would be worth whatever he would have to pay in terms of the bitterness that would inevitably ensue. The poem is brilliant in that it is able to present such deep-seated, seething emotions in such a simple form. It owes something to Petrachian conventions I suspect."

That night Dave phoned the author, John Barker, and indignantly informed him of this travesty. But he was even more indignant by the author's apparent blasé attitude to the whole thing. He remembered that the two of them had concocted the poem precisely for the purpose of sending up lecturers like Miss Morgan-Power. But as for going public and revealing to the world the preposterous nature of such interpretations, well he would have none of it.

"Surely you know the rules of the game by now?" he demanded of Dave. "Year after year candidates have sat down to answer questions about my poetry, about what it really means. You are the first one to actually ask me for my opinion and I am certainly not going to spoil things by telling the world, especially as this one was a spoof anyway. You will spoil the whole game if you are not careful. Do you want tutorials to last only five minutes instead of sixty? Do you want my poetry taken out of the set books altogether? No it is just not on."

"But it is so barmy." protested Dave. "The mild and bitter beer we were writing about have become epics. I could use all this in a little scheme I have to blow the gaff on this place."

"They will never believe you for a start. You are up against a system. And I won't back you up anyway. So if I were you I would forget it."

Chapter 12

The students at St. Brendan's had to be allowed some pranks or they would not have been proper students. The difference at St Brendan's was that the staff produced bigger and better pranks than the students. So it was that the skeleton sitting on the toilet in the ladies' loo was down to the students. The bubble car that mysteriously found its way up three flights of stairs and came to rest on the landing of a hall of residence was also down to the students. The case of Arthur Pitts was in a different category all together because of the implications it had for the college's relationship with the outside world.

It had all begun with a typical student stunt. When the register was sent round the large Education lecture groups the wags had grown tired of signing in Queen Victoria or Nelson so Dave had suggested the name of A.Pitts, short at the time for Arm Pitts but later for Arthur Pitts. The lecturer at the time of Arthur's birth was Frederick Stapleton, distinguished for a piece of research thirty years before and for a senility that had set in soon afterwards. He mistakenly called out the name of A.Pitts and it was promptly responded to in the affirmative.

Thereafter Pitts had a tick and so an identity. He was not struck off with Queen Victoria and Nelson. On the contrary, Matthew Brown sent him notes demanding to know the reasons for any absence. The jape snowballed and the more ambitious students produced elaborate variations on the same theme. Sometimes there was an uncomplicated refusal to answer his name so as to get him in trouble. They would then send a note of apology for his absence.

Sometimes they would send in essays on his behalf and get him noted as an average sort of student. As an experiment they had him reported to Matthew Brown's Progress Committee from which he received a deluge of Reminders, Remonstrations, Rebukes and the rest of Brown's armoury. In short they established an identity for him at a level lower than the general office which kept personal records but sufficient for him to count against student numbers and thus to attract a grant to the College. Arthur Pitts played for the Rugby team, was an official of the Students' Union, a paid up member of various societies and the fiancé of a girl in the third year.

Soon the joke had reached such proportions that his inventors began to reverse the process and cast doubts about his existence only to be shouted down by those who had supported him in the Union elections. The Thomist philosophers in the Theology Department, known as the God Squad, had even produced "Five Proofs of the Existence of Arthur Pitts". These were:

1. His name was on the lists and he regularly attended lectures.

2. Letters from and to him existed and bore his signature.

3. He was an Official of the Student's Union, elected by those who had a high regard for his abilities.

4. He played regularly for the Rugby team.

5. He was a member of the college library and owed it money.

It was the last one which was the clincher. Anyone who owed money was bound to exist because that money had to be paid back. Non-existence was not an excuse. It also caused a good deal of trouble all because the librarian had had an idea, a feat which was unusual in itself, but all the more unusual because he was able to retain it in his mind long enough to tell the Principal about it, but not much longer than that, because when the Principal brought it up again later he opposed it as unworkable and silly.

The idea had arisen because Arthur Pitts was a persistent defaulter who refused to respond to repeated requests to return his forty two borrowed books. Worse, rumour had it that he also stole books from the library. Sometimes the librarian quite liked people to steal his books. He was fond of saying that it showed that he was buying the right books. Sometimes he tried to think up ways of stopping this common practice. He decided to place in the spine of every library book, a metal strip which would activate an alarm if the book, concealed or not, was carried past a special detection device. The pre-operation trials worked well enough. Books legitimately borrowed were de-magnetised and those that were smuggled out were soon detected by the device. It was so successful that the librarian decided to have a grand opening ceremony to which the Board of Governors were invited. The actual ceremony was to take the form of the Chairman of the governors trying to take out a book without permission and being caught by the contraption at the door. He was duly caught red-handed but so were most of the other members of the official party because the machine provided incapable of distinguishing between the metal strips in the books and those in the gentlemen's braces. It also went on to be something of an embarrassment to quite a few ladies.

When these ladies fled to the toilet to adjust their bionic parts they were met by the unnerving sight of the skeleton which was a permanent resident of one of the cubicles. Arthur Pitts, fittingly enough was blamed both for the debacle in the library and the hysterics in the loo.

The skeleton had in fact been an unsuccessful attempt to unsettle Mrs Mason, also known as "Jodrell Bank", who lectured on Health Education. Being something of a pain in the neck herself she seemed quite suited to her role. She had health on the brain and her particular, if somewhat unusual, specialism was adult potty training. She had an educated ear for efficient toilet performance; she spied on staff by listening at doors and regularly ticked them off for inefficiency or inadequacy or impotence in this essential aspect of their lives. She could tell so much from the briefest of listenings that she had earned the nickname of "Jodrell Bank."

"Mr Jones," she once said to the mono-syllabic Art man, "I am not at all happy with the example you are setting for the younger members of staff in the matter of ... shall we say personal hygiene. May I remind you that when you perform your, er, necessity I should expect to hear certain noises such as the pulling of the handle, the flushing of the bowl and the running of the tap. It seems to me that you must be short-cutting some of these operations by pulling the handle before you have fully completed your business and thereby leaving the cubicle with a totally unnecessary health hazard to greet the next occupant. I also observe that your hands were not properly washed when you re-entered the Senior Common Room this morning."

"Sod off," was his predictable reply but it did nothing to solve the problem of Mrs Mason. She would prattle on undaunted through a whole series of such imperatives. She had once been a Health Visitor and true to her calling, she could spot a microbe at a thousand paces, kill it stone dead without its even knowing that it was within firing range and have it flicked into a plastic bag for safe disposal without even pausing in her conversation. She had plastered the notice boards with warnings against every known vice and health hazard and against some that were unknown to the students until she drew their attention to them. She weighed in against most forms of innocent amusement including visits to the local baths with the same degree of vehemence that she brought to recalcitrant abusers of toilets. Her opposition to the swimming baths brought her up against Mike Schofield who had a scheme for transporting students in his brother-in-law's minibus.

"How often do they change the water?" she demanded to know.

"Well you *should* know," was her answer to his confession of ignorance. "It might be all right at nine o'clock in the morning but what is it like in the afternoon eh? Tell me that." Then she remembered the fleas.

"Where do they put their clothes?"

"In the lockers of course. They are quite safe."

"They might be safe but are they clean? In my experience lockers are filthy, dirty places and full of fleas. I should feel it my duty to inform the Medical Officer of Health if my girls have to leave their clothes in flea-ridden lockers."

In desperation Schofield offered to ensure that the clothes would not go in the lockers but would be placed in neat piles on the benches in the changing rooms and not in the lockers at all. "How far apart?" was all he got for his trouble. Not only would it be a temptation for pickpockets but surely he knew the distance that modern strains of flea could be expected to jump, he being a P.E. man. She would want an assurance that the distance would be more than exceeded when the clothes were placed in piles.

It was inevitable that a brand of lavatory humour should have arisen around and about "Jodrell Bank" especially as everyone knew of her penchant for eavesdropping. Anyone who was ill would have duplicate stories to tell. The second would replace the words of ordinary discourse with more mysterious terms from medical books. She could then eavesdrop with relish, jump to horrific conclusions, advise people to make wills or take premature retirement or advise others to avoid them. The joke was considered to be doubly successful if it included gruesome details of toilet performance.

One thing led to another until the gang collectively responsible for Arthur Pitts placed a skeleton on a seat in the ladies' loo just off the library corridor. Once the initial fuss had died down it proved more difficult to remove than to put there. The cleaners would not touch it, the lady staff ignored it rather than remove it themselves, the men staff had no access to that particular room anyway and refused to go in. So it just stayed there as a monument to Mrs Mason and a frightener to new members of staff and to visiting governors as on the occasion of the grand opening of the detection device. It gave Mrs Mason the opportunity to come out with her one immortal line that toilets were dirty things and, if she had her way, she would not have them inside buildings at all.

The incident was blamed on Arthur Pitts but he could not be found and made to remove the skeleton because he was on teaching practice in a school. Even when enquiries proved that there was no-one of that name on the official lists the matter had to be handled carefully because, although he was not a registered student he had been included in the total numbers and the college had been getting a grant for him for the whole year. His departure from the college had to be handled without fuss.

He was not around to see Mike Schofield get his come-uppance over the matter of the coffee machine. It was difficult for a stranger to see how a simple, inanimate object such as a coffee machine could arouse such violent emotions but academics are strange folk, especially scientists who loudly proclaim that they are detached and objective because they have been trained to replicate other peoples' observations.

The seemingly inoffensive little object designed to bring some convenience into the lives of the assembled academics cast a blight on personal relationships and led to the demise of Mike Schofield's promising career as a wide boy. The Finance Officer had declared a cost-cutting exercise in which coffee breaks were abolished and catering staff deployed in other ways than serving drinks and biscuits morning and afternoon.

After the ritual deploring of his actions the staff debated the problem of irregular breaks and the provision of sustenance. The solution was thought to be in the provision of a coffee machine which would dispense coffee at all hours, need little attention, and be reasonably cheap to run. So far they had displayed nothing more than a touching faith in logic. They then made the fatal mistake of entrusting the provision of it to Mike Schofield who promptly looked to his brother-in-law who, he assured everyone, was one of the country's leading coffee importers. In no time at all Mike had fixed up the Senior Common Room Committee with a rental agreement on a coffee machine, or rather a five year rental agreement with a finance company which had paid him a substantial commission for the business. He had made a profit whilst they had a long term debt. As a result, the small annual fee to the Common Room, paid by all members of staff, was completely swallowed up by the rental debt and had to be increased.

Members had to pay an increased price for each cup of coffee. But when the original stock of coffee powder ran out, it was found that they could only re-order, and at exorbitant prices, from the rental company. Attempts to order from alternative companies foundered upon the small print in the contract. Consequently the price of each drink consumed had to rise regularly and often. Soon the staff had to solve a problem which would have taxed the most sophisticated medieval scholastic philosopher. The more they drank the more money they lost; the less they drank the less revenue they had to fill up the machine which they had to keep paying rental for anyway. General funds were already committed to meeting the rental so there was no possibility of a subsidy. Irate members demanded that the machine be sent back before they were all made bankrupt but again the small print prevented even this action. The machine represented a debt with a finance house which would remain irrespective of the location of the machine or its use.

A war of words ensued. Slogans appeared on walls:

"DRINK MORE," one would urge.

"DRINK LESS," said a counter sign.

"SEND IT BACK," was a simple plea.

"THE MORE YOU DRINK THE MORE YOU HELP."

"THE LESS YOU DRINK THE MORE WE SAVE."

Furious colleagues accused each other of drinking or not drinking as the case may be. Luddites threatened to break up the machine and vigilantes enrolled to protect it. Helpful, as ever, Mike Schofield suggested that they buy themselves out of the contract with the finance house for a lump sum and forfeit the machine in lieu of the rest of the debt. In order to do this the fees had to be put up by three hundred per cent. It was Mike's last venture at St Brendan's. He left on the same day as Arthur Pitts.

Chapter 13

Strange things were going on behind the doors of Committee Room B just off the main corridor of the teaching block of St. Brendan's. The College Academic Board was meeting. Committee work had become a disease of the brave new academic world and it was the bane of most sensible people's lives but others seemed to thrive on it. Moreover it tended to bring out the worst in people. One of Erfert's appointees had earned the nickname of "The Amendment-In-Search-of-A-Resolution," because of his objection to each and every proposition which came before the Board. Another one was the "Resignation Expert" because of his tendency to take offence at every minor criticism of himself. His most famous line had come in one meeting when he announced that; "Unless you withdraw that remark I shall be forced to resign."

"I certainly will not withdraw my remark," replied his opponent.

"Right then, if you are not prepared to withdraw the remark I am not going to resign." With that he sat back, confident that he had won some sort of a victory.

Dave listened to all this nonsense as the student representative. He did so as the result of an election, but the truth of the matter was that having fought for representation the students soon lost interest in the position and there was never anyone prepared to put themselves up for it. It was something of a hollow victory to be chosen but it suited Dave because it enabled him to see at close quarters the man he still wanted to expose and the system he was beginning to despise.

In Committee Room B there were a dozen or so highly paid academic staff, and a few others, deep in discussion about where to paint the white lines in the college car park and what to do about the ramps.

They had previously decided after long deliberation to build the most enormous ramps, or sleeping policemen, in order to make the traffic proceed more slowly through the campus. The fact that there had never been an accident in all the years of the college's existence played no part in the discussion but the fact that there was a sum of several hundred pounds left over at the end of the financial year did. The Health and Safety Officer was determined to get the Finance Officer to cough up the money and the latter had no real excuse for not spending and therefore risk losing the money from the funds. The trouble was that the ramps had been built at a height about three times that of a normal ramp and had effectively cut off the college from the outside world or at least to anyone who valued his exhaust. So now the discussion was about how to raise the roadway in order to bring it up to the level of the ramps. This was to cost thousands in an attempt to rectify the problem posed by the unnecessary ramps that had been built to spend a few hundred.

The second item of business was of interest to the student representative because it concerned the allocation of tutors to those students who were to go out into schools on Teaching Practice or T.P. as it was universally known. It was important not just because their teaching qualification depended upon it but also because some tutors were to be avoided at all costs. Because they never attended the Academic Board the students had always assumed that the allocation was done on a professional basis, taking account of the student, the location of the school, the subject to be taught and the specialism of the tutor. Dave was more than a little surprised to see the Principal diving into a bowler hat and matching up the names drawn with the student list held by the Registrar.

"Item three," said the Principal, "Evolution." Dave had not got a clue what that meant but he began to assume that it was the reason for the presence of the college Medical Officer who was sitting opposite him trying to look like a doctor even if he had forgotten most of the knowledge that went with the title. But before anything else could be said up popped the Amendment-In-Search-of-A-Resolution.

"I should like to move for an adjournment," he said.

"I will put it to the vote," replied Erfert.

"I object," protested the Resignation Specialist.

"You object to the adjournment?" asked the Principal.

"No, I object to putting it to the vote."

"Objection overruled," pronounced Erfert.

"How can you overrule it without first putting it to the vote? Besides I object to students being able to vote."

"Ok," said Erfert, "I will put to the vote the question of whether or not students can vote."

"If you put to the vote the question of whether

students should be allowed to vote, the student could be voting on whether he is allowed to vote. That would not be fair and I would have to resign."

"That might solve it,"said Erfert. "If you resign I might not have to put to the vote your suggestion that students should not be allowed to vote. Then we could vote on the substantive motion of whether we should put it to the vote or not."

"Right then, you have persuaded me that I should not resign but I want my objection to be minuted."

Dave could see that this could go on for hours for they seemed to be just warming up, so he gently made a suggestion. "Mr Chairman, would be helpful if I offered not to vote anyway?"

They were not used to people being helpful and were somewhat non-plussed by the suggestion. The objection specialist thought that it was probably unconstitutional for a person who may or may not be allowed to vote to waive the right or non-right, but in the end they did turn to the somewhat mysterious topic of "Evolution".

This turned out to be a row between the Science Department and the Religious Studies Department over the teaching of a common element in their courses; Evolution. The scientists were as unscientific as most academic scientists are in real life, taking refuge in assurances that they had been trained to think, rather than in anything resembling objective assessment of evidence. They accepted Evolution as a dogma to be believed without question and taught as a fact. They were happy to make huge unsupported generalisations about what happened millions of years ago and to draw nice neat charts of evolutionary developments with all the missing bits filled in for the sake of clarity. Where there was no evidence for their generalisations they wisely assumed, not that there was no evidence, but that it had not yet been found and when it was found it would fill out just what they had been confidently proclaiming all along. Even that might have been bearable if some of these scientists had not been Erfert's appointees, inferior men trapped in the prison of a single highly specialised discipline without vision, without proportion, without the correction of an educated mind; men who raised their single perspective to the status of an all-embracing explanatory principle for the world and all that lay therein; men who analysed poetry on a computer and regarded Arts men, and theologians in particular, as differing from scientists in that they were at an earlier stage of evolutionary development.

The staff of the Religious Studies Department were not much better. They were led by the ex-Jesuit who had abandoned his vows in favour of a literal interpretation of the Bible and a wife and family. His explanatory principle was just as simplistic as that of the scientists but slightly more flexible in that there was some room for a little argument here and there. God had created the world in seven days. He had created all the species independently and the species known as scientists had been something of a bad joke perpetrated by the Almighty in the aftermath of the Fall.

Whatever the reasons, these two departments were locked in a life and death struggle for the upper hand and for the minds of their joint students. They spent most of their time finding out from the students just what the other department had taught them about Evolution and countering

111

it before the students could be contaminated. The students had grown a little tired of playing piggy-in-the-middle and after the initial excitement of stoking up the furore by poetic licence, they had complained to the Academic Board, which is how it came to be on the Agenda. As in all such matters between furious academics, the personal animosities were rarely mentioned but were obvious to everyone though wrapped up in a cloak of rhetoric or pseudo-science. The two sides were asked to present their cases and the Board quite happily acted as judges of the Will of God at the Creation and/or the entire course of science since that time. It was obviously going to take them more than one session to solve this problem so there was in fact an adjournment as the Resolution-in-Search-of-an-Amendment had asked for in the first place.

The ex-Jesuit with the earring had spoken first. He stated his literalist view and added for good measure that only a scientist could seriously postulate that simple living cells could be formed spontaneously, out of nothing as it were, in some vague past when the right conditions were mysteriously formed, again out of nothing. Then he said the magic words; "The odds against that must be tremendous."

"Yes, they must, mustn't they?" mused Erfert who was always attracted to statistics. He turned to the Art man. "What kind of odds would you say would be involved in creating things out of nothing?"

"Ten to one,"came the prompt reply from the Creative department.

"Never," shouted the P.E. man.

"No, he is right," shouted a Sociologist.

112

"Doctor, what do you think?" Erfert asked of the medical man, who had dozed off.

"Oh, a lot, I should say," he said with all the confidence vital to a man of his calling.

By now the bidding was getting higher and higher and the odds increasing by the minute. Someone looked for a definitive statement from the Maths man who had been busily scribbling for the past ten minutes. He used his own specialism's way of bamboozling people.

"I would put it at one in ten raised to the power forty thousand," he said with just as much confidence as the other experts.

"There you are," exclaimed the Art Man triumphantly, "I told you it was about one in ten."

"I am sorry, I thought you were way out," apologised the P.E. man.

"Well that is it then," concluded the Principal who then went off into one of his disastrous mental meanderings.

"Tell me doctor," he said, "Where do transplants fit into all this?"

"Oh, a lot, I think," came the same confident reply.

"I only ask because transplants have changed an awful lot of things haven't they? Including Evolution. Men are walking around the streets today with other men's hearts and kidneys; soon it might be animal parts or spare arms and legs kept in a deep freeze to be used when required. It ought to affect how we evolve as a species but it also affects us at the Last Judgement surely. When we are all united with our earthly bodies are we to claim back all the bits and pieces that have been used by others? Are some of us going to get to Heaven by false pretences?"

The Board began to show great interest in these ideas but because time was running out even for them it was decided to ensure that the subject form part of the next agenda.

Chapter 14

Dave was thoroughly peeved by his experience at the Academic Board. It was beginning to dawn on him that he was in the middle not just of a game that was played on two levels but of a game within a game, a game as complex as those medieval representations of the heavenly spheres. It was not the kind of game that you could prepare for by running round the track until you dropped. Even if you recognised the idiocy of the whole thing there was still a sense in which the game had to be played. He himself had to decide whether to pursue what seemed a fruitless task of building up a dossier of all the absurdities he witnessed or to take the easy way out, be a good boy and enjoy himself at tax-payers expense.

The thing that puzzled him most was the attitude of the so-called sensible set. The students themselves were certainly not crackers, unlike most of Erfert's appointees. Some of the staff were sensible enough but no-one appeared to be interested in contributing to his dossier, a dossier which he knew would not be believed anyway by the outside world.

As an older person and a tax-payer himself, he had arrived at the College with some preconceived ideas about students but he had been wrong. He had taken it for granted that they would turn out to be dirty, scruffy, long-haired, weirdo's, prone to drug addiction, chronic laziness and perversions of various kinds. The girls would all be easy conquests, prone to sleeping around and probably militant feminists to boot. But they were not. His student colleagues were decent, hardworking, friendly people who accepted him at face value even though he had more money than they who were struggling on loans or grants that were reduced every year by the D.E.S. He had not told them about his previous job or about his intention to show up Dr Erfert although he never disguised his disgust at the Principal's antics. He was disappointed that the students seemed to be so apathetic about student politics and putting things right and seemed to be so tolerant of Erfert's private army of idiots. It would need a good deal of provocation to turn these students into the nasty band of militant activists of popular mythology. At St. Brendan's there was no such provocation. The students wanted a qualification. Dr Erfert was a nice man. He liked his students and they liked him. Dave liked him. He certainly did not fancy telling his friends about his real mission at St. Brendan's.

And then there was Jane. He was getting on famously with Jane but she did not really understand his animosity to Dr Erfert. Since the night of the baby-sitting they had grown ever closer and even Dave was coming to the view that this was girl worth marrying. Her Irish Catholicism was a drawback of course. She had had a strict upbringing; not that that worried Dave. He could even agree with some of her antipathy to modern permissive behaviour; indeed most of the students would. It seemed to be only the B.B.C. that thought otherwise. Most of the students were looking for stable relationships. They had the same abhorrence for the taking of life that Jane had but she seemed to hold such views with more tenacity than most. Mr Scott had given the girls the best advice they were to receive at St. Brendan's when he observed that nobody forced anybody to jump into bed with anybody else and the best form of contraception was the word "No". It was short and simple and was observed by almost everyone.

Having convinced the female students, Mr Scott had little problem with the males. On matters such as abortion, letting handicapped children die and Euthanasia for the old, the college was remarkably conservative. So what was the problem with Jane? Dave knew nothing about Catholicism and could not understand how central it could be to someone's life. Jane on the other hand could hardly contemplate the idea of marrying someone who was not a Catholic. Once married, he knew that she would be the most faithful of wives, a pearl beyond price, but getting her to accept a proposal in the first place was the difficulty. He for his part was not going to embrace her faith for all the wrong reasons and she would not want him to either. So matters dragged on in a desultory way for some time. Both parties were pretty miserable. In desperation, Dave consulted the ex-Jesuit, the man who advised the Principal himself from time to time, but all he got for his trouble was a diatribe against the Pope, who was, it appeared, an agent of International Marxism determined to ruin the church from within.

Matters were finally brought to a head when he became irritated by the fact that Jane was never able to go out on a Saturday night because, all of a sudden, she had something better to do. Jealousy made him follow her one night and he was surprised to find that she went to the local church. He was dismayed to discover that her increased visits had coincided with the arrival of a handsome, young Irish priest, and he thought the worst. He heard this only at second hand and he had no idea of what a friar was or what would be his relationship with his flock. He had never been in a Catholic church in his life and so his fears were compounded when he saw Jane disappear into a small cubicle, with a red light outside. He tip-toed to the door and gently opened it. To his great surprise and embarrassment he found his girl friend alone, praying to a grille in a wall and FOR HIM.

"Go away," hissed Jane.

"I beg your pardon," said the voice behind the grille.

"I am sorry Father," she said, "Someone from the College has just barged in" (she glared at Dave) "looking for me."

"Hold on, I will come out," said the priest, obviously aware that something odd was going on in his church.

"That's torn it,'' thought Dave, who now had decided to brazen it out. He was preparing to be at his truculent best but his timing was upset by the delay in the appearance of the priest. There was a good deal of bumping and scraping before another door opened and he entered, painfully propelling himself in his wheelchair. He was young and he was handsome; he was also the victim of motor-neuron disease. His double doctorate had been no safeguard against this. The pain-wracked face managed to smile at Dave's confusion.

"What can I do for you?" he asked.

"Er, I have come to see about getting married," stammered Dave.

Chapter 15

The College Academic Board had reconvened. The previous meeting, having failed to solve the problems of Evolution and getting into Heaven under false pretences, had adjourned to allow five sub-committees to give the matter further attention. Dave awaited their reports with some trepidation although he was certain that he would receive more ammunition for future use.

"Matters arising," announced the Principal, immaculate as ever in silver grey suit and matching tie.

"I have studied the Bible on the matters you raised last week, Principal," said the Head of R.E. "and I have come to the conclusion that you are worrying unnecessarily about unauthorised entry into Heaven. As you know, only one hundred and forty four thousand are going to get to Heaven anyway. If each century were to get its fair share of that total, it follows that the number of those with transplants will be statistically insignificant."

"Thank you," said the Principal. "In my opinion even one is statistically significant but we will let that pass and move on. Any more matters arising?"

"Yes, I would like to ask a question of the Religious Studies Department," said the scientist with the huge abdomen and a malicious glint in his eye. What he had to ask arose out of a hatred of the Head of R.E rather than from anything in the minutes. It took him a few minutes to settle himself in his seat for he sought to emphasise the importance of his question by grasping his huge abdomen with both hands and lifting its considerable weight on to the table in front of him.

"Are the members of the R.E. Department aware that some of their students, and one Jane Morgan in particular, have been praying to an assortment of saints in order to gain success in the examinations?"

"Yes, so what?" asked the Head of R.E.

"It is obviously an unfair advantage in that it is not open to atheists to do the same. They should pass the examinations on their own merits."

"Nonsense," said the Head of R.E.

"Yes, superstitious nonsense," said the scientist, turning round the word.

"Yes," roared the scientists.

"Resign," shouted the Resignation Specialist.

"Point of Order," shouted the Amendment- in - Search -of -a -Resolution.

Erfert had been listening carefully to the learned debate for it was the type of problem that interested him. It also appealed to his religious streak. "I can see some cause for concern here," he said. "We do not want to lay ourselves open to a charge of allowing an unfair advantage. We have our mission statement that says we treat everyone equally but it also says that we have to redress any disadvantage. I do not suppose that there are any saints that the atheists could pray to so it looks like a case where we will have to practise some sort of positive discrimination just like we do for the blacks, the elderly, women, foreigners, exchange students, the handicapped, the socially deprived, one-parent mothers, the unemployed, the recently bereaved and the rest."

"In other words everyone in sight," sighed Mr Scott under his breath. He tried to get the matter referred to yet another sub-committee but the thinkers on the Board would not be put off.

"Some of those saints were clever people, you know," opined Frederick Toser, historian, "Doctors of the Church and all that. I doubt if they would be much help in modern physics but they could certainly tip the balance in Religious Studies or in History and that sort of subject. I think that we should give this serious consideration, Principal."

"I suggest that we ask the Examinations Officer to compare the examination results of the Catholics and the Atheists over a five year period to see if there is any evidence of outside interference of the kind alleged," said Erfert.

"And what would you do if there was?" asked Dave who felt he ought to say something if only to defend Jane.

"I hope that you are not thinking of forbidding the Catholic students praying for success," warned the Head of R.E. "That would be unacceptable religious discrimination. I would refer you to the mission statement."

"No we would never do that," answered Erfert, reminded of what they did for Jews, Muslims, Sikhs, and Jehovah's Witnesses not to mention various cult members.

"Anyway they could cheat and pray extra hard in the period immediately before an examination or before the ban could take effect."

"I hope that you are not thinking of a mass conversion of atheists just before the examination either," snorted the scientist.

"No that would never do," said Erfert, not revealing that he had already had a large number of them vicariously baptised. "What we really need is some form of positive discrimination to make up to the Atheists what the Catholics may be getting out of their prayers to the saints. Of course it is always possible that we, like the Catholics, are deluding ourselves about the supposed benefits, in which case we need some sort of recompense to the Catholics for the time lost in praying when they could have been studying. Can we think of some way of bringing out the latent talent of the Atheists and using it to best advantage without the aid of saints?"

"What about Hypnosis?" said Dave, sarcastically. But his sarcasm was lost on this lot.

"Hypnosis, of course," exclaimed a delighted Erfert.

"Brilliant my boy. Why did not I think of that? The idea has tremendous possibilities. I really must congratulate you upon it. We all learn a great deal throughout our lives but we can only recall a fraction of it. If only we could hypnotise the Atheists we could perhaps get them to dig out all sorts of things from the subconscious and use it to advantage. Then they could not complain that the Catholics are getting any extra help."

Dave sat back, flabbergasted at the way in which his remark had backfired. Erfert's gang of cranks had left their seats to congratulate him on the brilliance of his idea. A dull, sickening sensation gnawed at his innards as he instinctively knew that there was more discomfiture to come. Someone suggested that the new system should bear the name of its originator.

"Good," said Erfert. "We can call it the 'Smithsonian Principle of Retrospective Kinetic Introspection.'"

Dave desperately tried to find a way out of this dilemma. The wart on his left cheek always wobbled when he was terrified and it was now bouncing up and down uncontrollably matching exactly the rise and fall of the science man's abdomen as it too bounced up and down on the table in excitement.

"Furthermore," went on the Principal to roars of approval from his team. "As it is your idea you shall have the honour of being the first student to be hypnotised. No, don't be modest about it. You have deserved it; hasn't he gentlemen?"

"Yes," roared the Erfert set. Even the sane ones supported the suggestion. They did not really approve of having students on the Academic Board and this was a way of getting even with the one student who seemed eager to attend.

Chapter 16

Dave received little encouragement from Jane when he recounted his story to her. His only hope was his father. He had put a call through to him earlier in the day and was eagerly awaiting a return call. It came through at last.

"Hello, Dave, I am sorry that I could not call you back earlier but I got tied up with a little item that would interest you. Before I forget, your mother wants to know if you are wearing your woollen socks. I'll tell her that you are anyway. She says that you are to change them everyday. I'll tell her that you do."

Dave was bursting to tell him about his latest experiences and launched into a non-stop tirade against Erfert and the Board and his present predicament. His father listened carefully to his tale of woe and then said, "So what is the big problem? I told you that you were banging your head against the wall anyway. Why can't you just forget about your crusade, sit back and enjoy yourself? I agree that it is all totally crazy but what is the worst that can happen? Some crank will come along and put you under, if he is lucky, and bring out some of the things that you learned long ago and have half-forgotten. Next week you will be laughing about it."

"I suppose so," said Dave doubtfully. "I can always use it in my dossier."

"I have got something well worth putting in your dossier. It is the thing I was telling you about. Have you heard of the Crombie Code? It is a redundancy package dreamed up by your pals at the D.E.S. It is a way of compensating large numbers of staff made redundant by the closure of so many colleges. Financially it is quite generous, especially for older staff who can retire on about two thirds of their present salary and they can get a lump sum as well. The pension part is index linked and they will save on travel and all that sort of thing. Quite a lot of people are looking forward to it."

"So what is remarkable about that," said Dave, "that scheme is only so generous because it was originally devised for civil servants and was offered to lecturers by mistake."

"The good bit is that, although it is generous and attractive, the people who get it are not actually retired and it is a condition that they have to keep applying for jobs and be available for any work that is offered to them."

"So?"

"So there are lots and lots of people applying for jobs that they do not want to get. All they want are rejection slips that they can send off to the D.E.S. so that they continue to get the Crombie money. A whole host of worried people send off applications for jobs, attend interviews and do their very best to scupper their own chances. Some have got it down to a fine art. They turn up drunk, or else show an awful ignorance of their subject, or they are wildly unrealistic in their applications. They apply to be vice-chancellors of universities and so on. They are as happy as Larry to get their rejection slip."

"It sounds daft all right," agreed Dave, " but what has it got to do with me?"

"From what I can gather these guys get their come-uppance at St. Brendan's. I have heard from several quarters that there is a real danger of Erfert appointing them, especially if they are ignorant."

Dave was not to know it but, just at the moment that his father was describing the system to him, a scene was being acted out in the Principal's office which would not have been out of place in Vaudeville.

"Come in, Come in," said Erfert to the scruffy individual who had presented himself as an applicant for the post of Principal Lecturer in Multicultural Studies. "Let me see, you were formerly a lecturer at Midhurst College weren't you?"

" Yes, Guv."

"Did you like it there?"

"No, Guv."

"Oh, Dear. Why ever not?"

"I didn't feel up to the job Guv. I am a bit long in the tooth to keep up with all that reading so the students tended to lose out especially when I began to flare up in lectures and assault some of the weaker ones. I thought that I had better tell you the truth about myself right at the outset so that I would not be wasting your time."

"That was very considerate of you," said Erfert thoughtfully. "Very kind indeed. But I think that you might be selling yourself short, you know. What was it that made you flare up? Can you put your finger on anything specific?"

"Well, I was pretty ignorant of my subject, and I am afraid it showed. The students knew more than I did and some of them took a great delight in demonstrating it. I then got worked up and there would be a confrontation."

If there was one thing that Erfert liked better than an admission of ignorance it was a situation of constructive conflict. To the astonishment of the would-be reject he assured him that; "We are all ignorant to a greater or lesser degree. Tell me about the conflict situation. What factors would you say contributed most to the confrontation?"

"Booze, mainly."

"Were the students prone to drink?"

"No, I was. I used to get boozed up every lunch time. It was the only way in which I could build up my courage to face the afternoon. I know that it shows me up in a poor light and that it has ruined my chances of getting a job here but I am grateful for you for giving me the chance to explain my problems and so I will leave you to get on with interviewing some more worthwhile candidates."

"Do sit down," said Erfert. "I think that you might be just the kind of candidate we are looking for. Can you give me an idea of the extent of the ignorance you say you have of Multicultural Studies?"

"I have to admit that my ignorance in that area is almost total," said the bewildered interviewee.

"Good," said Erfert. "Then we can make a start there. Can you tell me what you do not know about Gujerati?"

"Everything."

"Excellent. In fact you know enough about it to confidently assert that you know nothing about it?"

"Yes."

"So you see. You do know something about it after all. Now, would you say that the Levi-Straus theory was an essential part of the course as you would teach it?"

"No."

"Capital. What about Durkheim?"

"Who?"

"Durkheim."

"No."

"Good."

The poor man's eyes grew wider and wilder as it dawned on him that his little nest-egg was in danger of being snatched from him. "You mean that you like the answers I have given?" he asked in amazement.

"So far, I am quite happy with your replies," Erfert assured him.

"Then there was the heart attack I suffered last year," said the man in desperation. "I know that I omitted to put it in my application but I only concealed it because I thought it would count against me. I suppose that it will count against me now," he ventured hopefully. "It was a lie after all."

"A little one perhaps, but it shows that you really wanted the job here. I have to admire a man who knows what he wants and sets out to get it. It is something of a compliment to St. Brendan's that you were prepared to lie a little to come here. You might be just the type we want."

"What about my ill-health? I might die on you at any minute."

"What is it the Bible says? We none of us know either the day or the hour. You might live longer than I. Certainly we have all to go sometime. We can all be knocked down by the proverbial bus. Should we turn down your valuable contribution on the off chance that it might be a short-lived one? If you are worth appointing you are worth appointing; it is a simple as that."

The man was now in tears of desperation, wrongly assumed to be tears of gratitude by the amiable philanthropist. "Now, now," said Erfert. "No, tears, though they do you great credit. I think all the more of you for them. Take this note to the Bursar and tell him that you will be joining us in September. He will sort out the loss of your Crombie money and arrange for your salary and deductions etc to be resumed. No, don't thank me any more; just see the

Bursar and then phone your wife. She will be pleased that your are back in harness again, won't she? She will be able to make arrangements for selling the house and moving here. No don't try to thank me any more, really there is no need. I look forward to seeing you in September. For the moment good-bye."

Chapter 17

The Academic Board came to order. The Principal signed the minutes of the last meeting and dealt with matters arising.

"I have been informed by the Examinations Officer that there are some lessons to be learned from a comparison of the examination results of Catholics and Atheists but that the conclusions are not those that might be expected. It seems that, over the past five years, the top marks in Religious Studies have been gained by Atheists and that no student has passed Physics at the first attempt."

Dave jumped in very quickly at this point. "Oh, what a pity. But it was worth a try. I am sorry that it fell through but I suppose that the abandonment of our experiment at an early stage is better than getting to the middle of it before realising that we are on a false trail."

"Don't be so faint-hearted, my boy," said Erfert. "Who said anything about abandoning the experiment? It is a capital idea. If we have to reassess our premise we can still carry on with the second part of the scheme. That is why I have asked the distinguished hypnotist Professor William Bertrand to attend today's meeting. You are very welcome Professor. This is the young man who thought up the idea of asking you to improve the realisation of latent potential by tapping the barely remembered knowledge in the subconscious mind and who has volunteered to be your first subject in the college. He is very excited about it, as we all are."

The Professor was an egg-head in every sense of the word. His dome was completely bald and very elongated. His distinguishing feature was a pair of piercing blue eyes which flashed as he spoke to Dave.

"Now, Mr Smith, I want you to relax completely," he urged in a voice as soft as silk. "And when I snap my fingers you will feel very contented and you will be ready to answer my questions."

"Like Hell I will," thought Dave, struggling to retain control. But before he knew it not only he but also the scientist's large abdomen were completely asleep and motionless.

"What is your name?"

"Dave Smith."

"And you want to be a teacher Dave?"

"No," said Dave's subconscious.

"No?"

"No."

"But you are training to be a teacher are you not?"

"If you can call what goes on here, training."

"Don't you want to become a teacher then?"

"No."

"Then, why are you here?"

"I am here because I work for the D.E.S. and I intend to expose Dr Erfert and his precious College. He is a phoney and his college is full of loonies."

That was the end of that. After a few seconds of stunned silence all hell broke loose. Dave had succeeded in achieving the impossible. He had not only reversed the adulation of the loonies on the Academic Board to the point where they were vying with each other in trying to tear him limb from limb but he had also roused the sleeping giant of the smaller but very important party led by Mr Scott. If the first group were outraged by the perfidy of his attack on their hero, the second were aghast at the prospect of the outside world getting to know what went on at St. Brendan's. Their bread and butter was at stake. Even Mr. Scott saw at once that this particular student ought to be torn limb from limb. He also made a mental note to enlist the aid of the Principal's wife as he always did in crises of this kind. Come to think of it though, he had never encountered a crisis of this kind. His mind roamed over the college buildings and grounds. If they killed Smith could his body be hidden in an inaccessible spot? Would his demise cause more bad publicity for the college than would his exposure of Erfert? He decided that Erfert's good name was the most important thing. In any case that bloody man would probably insist on recording Smith's death in the minutes so murder had to be dismissed. Ah, well he could always take Crombie.

Others were not so calm. There were cries of "Kill the little swine," and "Keep the little bugger hypnotised for the rest of his miserable life,"ringing round the room. The Principal tried to speak but could not make himself heard and when he did he amazed everyone by appearing to be on Dave's side. First of all he asked the Professor to waken Dave. Dave was slowly aware of being stared at by twenty faces contorted with hatred and one face beaming with benevolence.

"I should explain to you Mr. Smith that my colleagues are somewhat incensed by your recent revelations under hypnosis."

"Yes, of all the low down, cunning, conniving, miserable little squirts…" contributed Dave's personal tutor in charge of his welfare.

"Let me continue," said Erfert. "As I was saying, you have informed us that you are some sort of undercover man for the D.E.S and that you are determined to denounce me as a phoney. I think that was the word you used."

"I should like to make a proposal," said the Amendment-in -Search-of-a-Resolution.

"What is it?" asked Erfert.

"That we chuck the little sod out on his ear."

"Do I hear a seconder?"

"Yes," roared nineteen voices. Even Miriam Woodstock had found a cause with which she could completely identify and she was bouncing up and down in her chair shouting,"Expel, Expel, Expel."

The Principal paused for a moment. Then he said; "Well, I suppose we shall have to vote on it. Is anyone willing to defend Mr Smith as is his right?"

"NO!" was the universal shout.

"It would usually fall to you wouldn't it?" asked the Principal of the Head of Pastoral Care.

"No thank you. Wild horses on their bended knees would not get me to defend that little creep."

"A colourful image to be sure," replied Erfert. "Well, as his only supporter in the room, I suppose that his defence will fall to me."

A stunned silence greeted this statement. Then Mr Scott stammered in disbelief, "You surely do not mean that you are going to defend him after what he has said about you?"

"Certainly."

"But it makes no sense. He is out to ruin you; and all the rest of us if it comes to that."

"Yes, I accept that that is his intention. But he has an investigation in hand with which I have some sympathy. He formulated an hypothesis about me whilst he was in London and he has designed a research experiment to test it out in the field. It reminds me of the time when I had to resort to the subterfuge of being the college gardener for a while in order to facilitate my investigation into college groups and sub-groups without the problem of my own intrusion into the situation. I think that Mr. Smith may have a promising future as a social scientist and that his project may well be counted as a final year project. I certainly think that he should have the chance to complete it. And consider this. If I help him and if he can convince me of the validity of his conclusions I am prepared to sign his work as being valid and reliable. There are not many research topics that can claim that sort of endorsement."

"But surely to God you cannot be expected to actually help him to show you up?"asked the desperate Mr Scott. "How can we chuck him out or send him to Coventry, or kill him, if you are the only one on his side?"

"That would pose a problem all right but I think that the credibility of the research is a higher good."

Mr. Scott began to think frantically about some of the usual dodges in his damage limitation locker but none seemed to suit this bizarre situation. Then the sight of the doctor dozing away across the table from him gave him an idea. The doctor was dreaming peacefully about his days in Bombay as a medical student, when he had been told that he had not passed well enough to practise in the sub-continent but why did he not try Britain?

"Dr.Meredith," said Mr. Scott but there was no response from the doctor. "Dr. Meredith," he repeated and the doctor shot up, reached for a pad in front of him and wrote out a prescription for Librium. Mr Scott tried for a third time. "Dr.Meredith could you answer this question for me? Have you heard enough today to convince you that this young man is in need of psychiatric help on the grounds that he is obviously unstable?"

"I certainly have,"said the doctor. "Which young man are you referring to?"

"That one there with the wrong shaped temples and ears."

"Oh Him. Yes he definitely needs to see a psychiatrist. I will arrange it if you like."

"Thank you very much doctor. I thought he would not escape your professional sharpness. There you are Principal. I think that we can resolve this matter without resorting to a formal trial or asking you to be put in the invidious position of defending the wretch. The lad needs help not punishment. If his conclusions ever see the light of day, and I hope they will not, they will be discounted by all who know his background and if you sign his conclusions, as you seem determined to do, it will appear to one of your well known acts of generosity and care for the welfare of your students."

"Can't we declare him to be insane now and just get the psychiatrist to confirm it?" demanded Toser who knew of many instances in History by way of precedents.

"No it would be better to do it the other way round," smoothed Mr Scott who was feeling quite pleased with himself now. He knew that Dave was right but he could not let him blow the gaff on Erfert. Too much was at stake. He certainly could not let Erfert loose on the verification of Erfert's own looniness. Nor could he let the Board lynch Dave as they obviously wanted to do. The sight of him lying there in the chair, obviously drained of all life touched his not very touchable heart.

Declaring him to be insane was letting him off relatively lightly in Scott's opinion. Besides, he had it in mind that it would be only a temporary illness; he would soon recover but his original malady would remain on file in case he ever tried to denounce the Principal in public again. It was not the only time that Mr Scott's dexterity was to save Dave Smith.

Dave went back to his room and locked the door. There was no telling what enemies he had made and what they might do to him. His first thought was to pack his bags and make a run for it before the story got around. He would have to send for his heavier items and he had no time to dismantle his C.B. He would stay in his room until nightfall and then creep down without saying a word to anyone and be off before the inevitable student lynching party could be formed. It did not work out that way however. In a very short time he heard the sound of heavy feet thudding up the stairs leading to the room and raised voices that sounded very angry and then came the rat-tat-tat of angry fists on his door.

"Come out you rat," bellowed a he-man voice. "We know you are in there."

Dave looked desperately round the room for somewhere to hide. In a room measuring nine feet by twelve and containing regulation student amenities, there was not much scope for ingenuity. He had a bed, a bookcase-cupboard and a sink. The door proved no match for the beefy crew pitting their strength against its flimsy lock. It burst open under the combined weight of two hefty girl hockey players and several members of the first eleven who had never forgiven him for his training sessions and who now had the opportunity to work off their aggression with the backing of the whole college. When they had finished with him Dave was left trouserless and dishevelled in the College Quadrangle, staggering this way and that, half blinded by the St.Brendan's version of tarring and feathering which featured Marmite and Cotton Wool buds. Only the flap of his old fashioned woollen shirt stood between him and a charge of indecent exposure.

After some moments of panic and mental confusion he gradually became conscious of the fact that the angry crowd had melted away and he took the opportunity, since he was on his knees anyway, of offering up a prayer to St. David for his release from their torment. Then, doing a passable imitation of Groucho Marx's famous low walk in an effort to keep the flap of his shirt as low as possible, he half- ran and half-crawled into two pairs of shiny, brown, expensive looking shoes. The one pair belonged to Dr.Erfert and the other to a distinguished looking stranger who seemed to take more than a passing interest in Dave's strange antics.

"Excuse me," mumbled Dave through a mouthful of evil tasting cotton buds. "I must go and clean up."

"Are you aware that you are not wearing your trousers young man?" asked the stranger.

"Oh, yes," answered Dave, sarcastically. "I come out here every night dressed like this and pray to St. David."

"And why do you do that?"

"Because I'm nuts; didn't you know?"

"He is not really mad of course," volunteered the Principal. "He has just had a trying day."

"Oh yes I am,"shouted Dave. "The Academic Board said I am, the students said I am, and I say I am, so I must be."

"But what makes everyone think that you are mad?" asked the stranger.

"Well you see," said Dave conspiratorially, "I am a sort of special agent on an undercover mission. My job was to be as inconspicuous as possible and ..."

"You don't look very inconspicuous," interrupted the stranger.

"Ah, that is because I am auditioning for a part in the Desert Song," snapped back Dave in his usual unfortunate way.

"Yes, of course," said the man reaching for a notebook. "Now can you explain to me just what you hope to achieve by spying inconspicuously, dressed in a night-shirt, in the quadrangle and praying rather loudly to St.David whilst preparing for a part in the Desert Song."

"Certainly," said Dave, "not that it is any business of yours. I intend to prove that Dr. Erfert is a phoney who is doing harm to hundreds of students, that he has filled this College with a crazy gang of like minded loonies and that when I tell my story to the D.E.S. they will have to believe me and close this place down.." Having said this he gathered up his garment and, with as much dignity as he could muster, he made off, knees bent, back to his room. He was followed by Erfert and the stranger who seemed to be taking an inordinate interest in his predicament. They caught up with him as he reached his door.

"I see that your door is badly splintered. How did that happen?" asked the stranger.

"Mice," said Dave.

"Mice?"

"Grown up mice."

"Tell me young man. How well do you get on with your mother?"

"She is trying to smother me."

"And how does she try to do that?"

"With woollies; socks and jumpers and cardigans and gloves."

"But surely you are safe enough here. She cannot get you here."

"Oh can't she? Just have a look in that cupboard."

The man opened the cupboard and was promptly engulfed by hundreds of the said items. "But these must have cost a fortune. Can she afford to smother you?"

"She hasn't paid for most of them. She gets them free at Tesco's. Lots of people contribute to the smothering fund."

The man looked at Erfert and tapped his head meaningfully. "And what does your father say about all this?"

"He thinks I am mad too."

"So everyone thinks you are mad including yourself and your father. In fact the only person who thinks you are not mad is the one you think is mad."

The psychiatrist turned to Erfert and said, "I am glad you brought me in so quickly. Who knows what might have happened if you had delayed. It looks like a classic case of mother-fixation. He is obviously a Kleptomaniac with a passion for woollens and now he thinks that his mother is trying to kill him. Probably she did try to smother him in his cot and he dimly remembers the experience. Now he is transferring the fixation to your good self and thinks that his problems will be solved when the world agrees with his preposterous suggestion that you are a phoney. His father is in the role of the world in all this, in other words the world that still has to be convinced, the world that thinks he is mad. He is sane enough to know that others think him mad so the solution to his problems will in fact only come when he realises that the world is right to think him so. Instead of fighting it he must accept the verdict of everyone else. Only when he really assents to the proposition that he is mad will he be sane again."

"Would it be better for him if we asked him to leave?"

"It would be most imprudent for him to go anywhere at the moment. The world that is important to his fantasies is right here and the solution is right here. It was very perceptive of you to play the part of the only one who thinks he is sane when he thinks you are mad. We can use that."

Dave listened to the last part with the dawning realisation that he should be alarmed not flippant or sarcastic. He was about to try to explain the situation when the C.B. radio crackled into life. "One-four for a copy," said a voice.

"Caveman receiving you," said Dave automatically.

"Hello Caveman. This is Doctor Death calling to see if you fancy and eyeball. By the way, was it you that got rid of Arthur Pitts? Not before time if you ask me. He was getting to be a pain."

"My God," said the psychiatrist, "We have uncovered a whole nest of them."

Chapter 18

They left Dave lying on his bed, sobbing into his cotton wool buds and employing a vocabulary that even he never knew he possessed. He was too distressed to answer his C.B. callers. He was too marmited to leave the room even if the porter on guard at the door would have let him. The psychiatrist had promised to visit him on the morrow for a "chat", and Erfert had very kindly renewed his offer of help to denounce Erfert to the world. The outlook did indeed look bleak and the antics of Alun Evans the Welsh student who lived next door did not help. It was Evans' life ambition to convert all the students on his floor to his own fiery brand of socialism and he was at this very moment subjecting everyone to the speeches of Nye Bevan played at full volume on his record player. In desperation Dave turned to his C.B. and used the emergency channel to summon up help.

"Hello, hello, Caveman calling Dr. Death. Come in Dr. Death. This is an emergency, repeat, this is an emergency."

"Hello, Caveman, this is Vampyra calling. It is a long time since I heard from you. What have you been up to you naughty boy?"

"Look Vampyra this is an emergency. Can you help me out?"

"Of course I can, anything for you," she purred seductively.

"Hello, Caveman, this is Dr.Death here. I got your message but Vampyra cut in on me. What can I do for you?"

"This is Vampyra here. Clear off Dr. Death. I was the first to offer help so just clear off."

"Clear off yourself. You might have been the first to offer help but I was the first that he asked for help so clear off yourself."

"He has just this minute asked me for help. Isn't that right you lovely boy?"

"Yes, that's right Vampyra but ..."

"Keep out of this Caveman. This is between me and Vampyra. Look, you superannuated siren, what kind of emergency service are we running if you cut in and insist on helping people who don't want your help?"

"What kind of help are you giving Caveman by insulting me. He distinctly asked me for help. You don't even know what his problem is. Go on tell me what his problem is. You can't can you? No, you can't. Admit it you don't know."

"Of course I don't know. You cut in before he could tell me. For all I know he could be lying on the floor with a broken leg. Anyway, come to think of it, you don't know what is wrong with him either so why don't you just get off the phone and let me help him?"

"Look folks," began Dave.

"Don't interfere, Caveman. I am not letting this two-bit Jezebel with a cheapo rig tell me what I can and cannot do. She has not been on the air more than a few weeks and she thinks she can boss me about."

"Who says my rig is a cheapo?"

"I do."

"Prove it."

"I don't need to prove it. It is obviously a twenty quid job from Comet."

Dave decided to switch off; there would be no help forthcoming from the emergency channel. If only one of them would shut up he could get them to phone his father. He would know what to do. Otherwise he had visions of spending the rest of his life imprisoned in his little cell, guarded day and night, totally misunderstood and growing more and more mad as Erfert helped him to undermine Erfert. He spent a largely sleepless night dreaming of the Count of Monte Cristo and the Man in the Iron Mask both being tortured in turn by Dr Erfert.

In the event it was the psychiatrist who turned up to torment him.

"Look," said Dave, "I know that what happened yesterday will take some explaining but I want you to know that there is a perfectly simple explanation for the whole thing. You see I was attacked by a group of students who had a grudge against me ..."

"Do a lot of people have grudges against you?" interrupted the psychiatrist in his most soothing voice.

"Well there are one or two who have taken a dislike to me recently but I am sure that when I explain to them that..."

"One or two ?"

"Well maybe forty or fifty."

"Forty or fifty ?"

"Well forty or fifty staff "

"And the students?"

"I suppose that might be a few hundred more but..."

"Some people must like you though?"

"Of course."

"Can you name any?"

"Not off hand."

"A girl friend perhaps?"

"She isn't speaking to me at the moment."

"I SEE." There was a wealth of meaning put into the word.

"What do you see?" demanded Dave.

"What do you think I see?" countered the quack.

"You think I'm nuts don't you ? But I am not. A lot of people have taken a dislike to me but it is just temporary. I've upset a few apple carts because this place is a madhouse, run by a lunatic, but it suits some people to put up with it."

"So you are the sane one and all the rest are mad?"

"Not all of them. Most of them."

"Especially the Principal?"

"Especially the Principal."

"What about Mr Scott?"

"Oh, he is not mad. He knows what is going on all right."

"But isn't he the one who first suggested that you needed treatment?"

"Yes but he only did that to prevent me from revealing to the world just what is going on here."

"So most people are mad. Most people also think you are mad. One of the sane ones also thinks that you are mad."

"Yes," said Dave.

"Have you ever thought that there might be a simple explanation for all this?"

"No. What might that be?"

"That you are mad."

"Oh, go to Hell," shouted Dave at the top of his voice.

"Before I do that could you just help me put a few of these blocks of wood together so that they make up a shape?"

"No I could not," snorted Dave, "if you want them put into shapes why don't you buy them already in shapes?"

"I did. I took them apart before I came."

"And why did you do that?"

"So that you could put them together again."

"More fool you. That doesn't sound very sensible to me."

"Oh well," sighed the psychiatrist who did not quite know how to proceed in the event of someone refusing to do his test. He took refuge in scribbling furiously in his notebook. Then he said hopefully; "I don't suppose you would like to do a word association test?"

"No."

"A personality test?"

149

"No."

"A blot test?"

"No."

"Why don't you like your mother?"

"Who said I don't like my mother?"

"You did."

"I did not."

"Yes you did. You said that she tried to smother you when you were a baby."

"I most certainly did not. I said she tried to smother me by sending me loads and loads of woollens to wear."

"And you resent that?"

"No."

"But you don't wear them. You have a cupboard full of them. You cannot bring yourself to wear anything that woman has sent you can you? You dislike your mother don't you?"

"I don't like her sending me all those woollens. She embarrasses me. But I don't dislike her."

"Don't you think that she looks like Dr Erfert?"

"She is nothing like him. Apart from being a woman, she is tall and he is small and bald-headed."

"But there is a resemblance?"

"No."

"What about your father?"

"What about him?"

"Has he said that he thinks you are mad?"

"Yes but that is just a turn of phrase."

"Phrases tend to represent thoughts?"

"No, You have got it all wrong. He said that I was mad to take on the Educational establishment and the D.E.S."

"Isn't he right?"

"I am beginning to think so."

"I ought to tell you that I rang the D.E.S. this morning and they say that you asked to be sent here and because you had been acting rather strangely in the office they agreed to your coming here in the hope that you would recover your senses."

"How was I acting strangely?"

"I don't know the full story but it had something to do with a suggestion box that you were misusing and colleagues that you were insulting. Now tell me about Arthur Pitts."

"What about him?" asked Dave suspiciously.

"He is one of your friends isn't he?"

"Er, yes, in a manner of speaking."

"Does he think that you are mad?"

"No."

"Are you sure about that?"

"Positive."

"Good, then all we have to do is to get him to testify to that effect."

"I doubt if he will do that. He has gone away."

"That is unfortunate. Do you know where we can get in touch with him?"

"I wouldn't know," said Dave defensively.

"But I thought that he was a friend of yours."

"So he was."

"WAS?"

"I mean IS . So he is."

The psychiatrist suddenly leaned forward and slammed his notebook on the desk. "Where is Arthur Pitts? What have you done with Arthur Pitts? You were his friend. You were the last to be in touch with him. You were able to tell the Principal about his Baptism. Yet you still say that you know nothing about his whereabouts. That will not do. It seems that you were the last person to see him ALIVE."

He had now dropped his friendly manner and smooth voice. He was now convinced that he was dealing with a murder investigation. Dave, for his part, was convinced that he was dealing with yet another expert loonie and began to be frightened of being alone with him. He thought it best to cool things down.

"I have a confession to make," he began.

"Ah, you murdered him. I knew it."

"No, I did not murder him. The fact is Arthur Pitts never really existed."

"What do you mean; he never really existed?"

"Well I sort of made him up. He was a figment of my imagination. Then I sort of killed him off. But it was not murder. I just killed off my own creation."

"My God, this is an interesting case," cried the psychiatrist. Creating an imaginary friend and killing him off was text book stuff. He was all the more convinced when Dave suddenly turned to the blank wall and roared at the top of his voice that he was also going to murder Aneuran Bevan as well.

Chapter 19

Dave's state of mind was steadily deteriorating. He was isolated from the rest of the college. He could get no help from his C.B. Jane had made no move to get in touch and bribery had failed to remove the porter from the door. The police had been called into solve the mystery of Arthur Pitts and they too were in grave doubt as to whether he had been murdered by Dave or had been invented by him as a part of his obvious madness. Dave might have been able to withstand these pressures if it had not been for Erfert's visits to help him build up a dossier against Erfert himself. Not only was he a mine of first hand information but he started from the premise that Dave was right and proceeded to build up a better case than Dave could ever have done.

Dave thought long and hard about how he might get out of this nightmare situation. The only thing that he could come up with was to demand to see a priest (but not the ex Jesuit in charge of the R.E Department). No one ever refused a condemned man the right to spiritual solace and the Franciscan at the local church struck him as being an eminently sensible man. Furthermore it might get him out of his room, for the cripple could hardly be expected to climb up all those stairs. He was also a link with Jane and he might prove to be a link with his parents who were as yet ignorant of the plight of their son. Part of his problem was after all, the evil intent of his mother.

And so it was that a solemn procession made its way down the drive to the church. A porter led the way and he was followed by Dave and Dr Erfert. A second porter brought up the rear. Malevolent faces peered down from the windows and followed them all the way.

Dave stumbled into the priest's living room. He had no idea what kind of reception he would get, especially after the unfortunate circumstances of their last meeting but he need not have worried. Fr Terence had greatly deteriorated since he had last seen him. Then he had been able to wheel his own chair, now he had to be pushed into the room by another priest. He apologised for his weakness not fully appreciating that it was a source of great spiritual uplift to those to whom he was a burden. He was not quite strong enough to take the tale that Dave blurted out in a torrent of words exuding self pity and a confused state of mind.

"Calm down," he begged. "Take a breath and start again. I have all the time in the world to listen to you and I am very glad of your company for as long as you can stay." He did not look as if he had all the time in the world. His voice was weak, his cheeks were gaunt and his hands lay gnarled and lifeless on his lap. But his Irish eyes still contained the twinkle of good humour that had characterised his personality throughout his life. Dave stopped in full flood and realised for the first time that he was looking at a happy man. How could such a man, burdened by far more troubles than Dave was, be so composed and tranquil in the face of Nature's cruel strokes?

And so it was that Dave launched into a slower more lucid version of his tale of woe, including the obvious comment that he did not expect Fr.Terence to believe him anymore than the rest did. He went through the whole story, from the D.E.S to the madhouse at St. Brendan's, to his troubled relationship with Jane and the mind-blowing lunacy which lay at the heart of a so-called respectable science called "Education". What should be a vital part of every child's inheritance seemed to be a meaningless mish-mash of pseudo- scientific and pseudo-sociological clap-trap in an academic environment which seemed to tolerate any zany theory and seemed incapable of even recognising, let alone dealing with, idiots like Dr.Erfert. He was not even inhibited by the presence of the smiling Dr Erfert helping him out with some of the more difficult words.

"Bravo, well done," said Erfert when he paused for breath.

"And they are preventing me from seeing my parents. Do you think you could phone my father for me?" he pleaded.

"I am afraid I cannot do that," said the priest, but he got no further before Dave's well known impatience got the better of him, accusing him of being like all the rest, of not believing him and of being taken in by so called experts like the psychiatrist.

"Hold on," said the priest, "I did not say that I would not phone him. I said that I could not phone him. It is my hands you see. They do not do as they are told anymore. I cannot hold the receiver but if you wish to phone your father yourself by all means do so. I will speak to your parents myself if you will hold the phone for me."

A thoroughly embarrassed Dave wondered what it was about him that made him produce hasty, foolish, unthinking comments such as he had just come out with. No wonder people were against him. No wonder people thought him mad. In the event, his father was phoned and put in the picture and between them they agreed to accept the priest's kind invitation to stay at the presbytery instead of returning to his place of torture. His father would drive up as soon as possible to try to sort it out. A great weight had been removed from Dave's mind and, curiously, a great deal of comfort was gained just by being with the pain-wracked figure opposite who had been the only one to listen to him without interruption and the only one to make the slightest effort to help him. When he did speak Fr Terence produced a practical list of things to be done.

"I suggest that three things be done. First let your father worry about a strategy to get you out of this mess. Secondly allow me to get Jane down here so that we can sort out your love life. Third, when you have had something to eat and when you have removed some of that black stuff from your face, we will have a long talk about Education, Erfert and anything else that you care to raise."

"I doubt if you will be able to understand what I am on about unless you know something about Education. It is a bit like a cult; it is difficult to understand unless you have been subjected to it yourself."

"Try me," said the priest, smiling as his eyes looked at the picture on the wall behind his young detractor, a picture of a young cleric loaded with degrees and an academic career so distinguished as to embrace Cambridge and Rome and professorships in Philosophy and Theology. He spared Dave any further embarrassment by not mentioning it. It was not the practice of religious orders to parade individual achievements like the exotic plumage of some of Erfert's appointees did. Instead he said; "If you are to marry Jane you will need a few talks about her religion, not to convert you, you understand, but to help you to realise what her religion means to her. Then there is the bringing up of children, and that brings us back to Education again. It might be that a proper appreciation of her religion will help to put your academic problem in perspective because there are many false gods in the temples of Education, especially in this country."

Settled in the old leather armchair talking to a calm, sensible and serene man made Dave forget his troubles for a while and he started to chat away about the Catholic religion as he knew it. That is to say he produced a lot of misconceptions and folk lore which the priest had heard a thousand times before but was too polite to contradict. Dave found to his surprise that, however frail might be his body, there was nothing wrong with his new friend's mind. He soon had the warm sensation of being in touch with real academic quality of a kind that was absent from St. Brendan's. He was fascinated to find that the Irish-educated young man had gone on to study in a broad European tradition; Theology and Philosophy in Rome and Paris through the medium of Latin or French or Italian as the case may be, History at Cambridge and lectureships in several institutions until his order sent him to the United States and finally to an obscure little parish in England at the onset of his crippling affliction.

"Did you not miss the academic high life?" asked Dave, unable to credit someone with willingly taking a step down from the ladder of success.

"I go where I am told and I do what I am told," was the simple reply.

"How come?"

"Because that is my vocation and my choice. And who is to say that helping the ordinary people of this parish is less worthy than lecturing to the brightest youngster in the land?"

It soon turned out that here was a man who had a completely different version of everything that Dave had ever taken for granted. He had a sort of medieval view of an educated man; a man not in the prison of his own narrow specialism but a man of all-round achievement with some vision of what the world was about and how his bits of knowledge fitted in with a wider view of things. Dave contrasted this in his mind with the misfits who taught him a vast number of seemingly unrelated disciplines and so-called sciences. With growing excitement Dave began to think of him as someone who could make some sense of his own life as well as helping him to overcome his present problem. He asked question after question until the priest's physical condition made it imperative for him to retire for the night. Dave, however, made no move to go up to his room but stayed up all night excitedly thinking up bigger and better questions to put to him on the morrow.

When dawn broke on the following morning he was up bright and early despite his lack of sleep. As the sun came up with the promise of a splendid morning he whistled a little tune to match that of the birds outside the window and he waited for his mentor. He was disappointed to hear the sound of the wheelchair approaching and then passing by the sitting room.

"First things first," Fr Terence explained later. "A priest's first job is to say Mass and that is what I do every morning before I have my breakfast."

"Can't you have a lie in then?"

"Not as long as I can make it to the chapel." That gave Dave a few more questions to add to his growing list.

In the event a couple of callers arrived to interrupt further explanations. The first was Jane who was ushered into the sitting room by the housekeeper and found to her surprise Dave in deep conversation with her friend.

Fr. Terence at once turned on a little Blarney to cover her embarrassment and raised a smile as she answered him in a similar vein. With a bit of mental dexterity the priest went on to prove that she had been an accessory-before-the-fact since Dave had confided in her some time ago about his intentions towards Erfert. Was it really fair now to brand him as a traitor, a fifth columnist, a Quisling?

After a while he coaxed her into admitting that perhaps she had been too hasty, and into promising that she would try to help Dave if he would stop persecuting poor Dr.Erfert. Dave bit back his response and felt all the better for so doing.

Jane was particularly helpful in that she could give him the news about the latest state of play at the college. The police had found the skeleton sitting on the toilet seat in the ladies and were trying to identify it as that of Arthur Pitts. The Health and Safety Officer had declared himself determined to smell gas in any room occupied or likely to be occupied by Dave Smith and the Bursar had actually agreed to corroborate the same.

The students as a body felt betrayed by Dave. They were not disposed to declare him insane but hated him with an intensity that had to be seen to be believed. Mr Scott had consulted Mrs Erfert on the best ways to get him off the hook and Dr. Erfert was taking round a petition on his behalf. His son Brian, however, and given evidence to the police that he had been viciously assaulted by Dave when the latter had been babysitting some time earlier. It was at that point that Dave's mother and father arrived.

His father came with the family G.P.and a plan. His mother arrived with a box of woollens which she insisted on giving to the priest to keep warm his aching joints.

The family physician looked at Dave through his bi-focal spectacles and reminded him that having brought him into the world he did not really expect to have to follow him through it in order to look after his every need. That, he reminded him, was not the meaning behind the term "family doctor."

"I am sorry to cause everyone so much trouble," stammered Dave, "but your professional opinion might prove to be valuable at the moment, and you have known me all my life. What do you think of my state of mind?"

"I think you are mad."

"What!" gasped Dave.

"I think that you are mad to think that you can possibly take on the whole educational establishment and hope to get away with it. You might not be insane but you are crackers just the same."

"Thank God for that," said Dave, much relieved. "But what about the psychiatrist. He is supposed to be an expert and he thinks I am mad."

"That is another reason why I think that you are mad. How you ever let yourself get into the clutches of one of those guys, I will never know. No self respecting doctor would make that mistake."

"I promise that I won't make that mistake again," said Dave with feeling. "But how am I going to get out of this one?"

"The best way to deal with experts is to get another expert to give a second opinion. For a fee you can get an opinion on anything. The courts are full of experts contradicting each other and so is my profession. They hate it and love it at the same time. Its part of a game. It so happens that your father's union has a tame psychiatrist who specialises in counselling those teachers who have broken down trying to be pastoral care teachers in secondary schools."

"And if that doesn't work?"

"If that does not work we will decide that you have only temporarily gone off the rails because of some drugs that I put you on to cure a mild complaint. We can effect a cure by taking you off them."

"If you do rehabilitate him it will only open him up for prosecution," said Jane. "Most of the staff hate him, most of the students will not talk to him, and the police might charge him with murder if he is not insane. The psychiatrist is talking about operating on his frontal lobes because he is not fit to plead."

"There is one thing the psychiatrist said to Erfert that might be of help," said Dave desperately. "He said that I would not be considered sane until I admitted that I was mad and that everyone else is right to think me mad. Can you make anything out of that?"

"I think that I should have a word with this psychiatrist fellow," threatened his mother.

"Oh, no, don't do that," urged Dave imagining the disastrous consequences of such an encounter. "He thinks that you are the cause of the whole thing in the first place. He has got it into his head that you tried to smother me in my cot and that the traumatic experience has unhinged me to the point where I have transferred my hatred of you to Erfert. That is why I am trying to ruin him. It is all very confusing I am afraid."

His mother then stunned him by saying thoughtfully "I wonder how he knew what happened so long ago."

"Right, that's it then,"said the doctor. "Your mother goes to see the psychiatrist demanding help because she is going to make a second attempt on your life. He is as pleased as Punch that his reading of the situation is correct. You go to see him and tell him that you have come to accept that you really are mad. He assures you that he has got to the root of your problem and counsels you to forgive your mother and not transfer her guilt to Erfert. I get the union psychiatrist to give a second opinion that agrees with the first one so everyone ends up trying to persuade you that you are sane against your own insistence that you are mad. You are released from your evil spell and the shrink goes back to play in his darkened room."

"BRILLIANT", shouted Dave, punching the air with his fist.

"But what about the police?" demanded Jane.

"Oh, I am sure that you can round up enough sensible students own up to the truth about Arthur Pitts and the skeleton in the loo."

"Maybe I could," she said doubtfully. "But let me warn you Dave Smith. If you ever get out of this scrape in one piece you will never, repeat never, get into this sort of trouble again. How can I marry Public Enemy Number One?"

It took Dave some moments to grasp what she had just said but when he did so he leaped from his chair with a great yell of delight. The sun beamed all the brighter and there were big hugs all round.

Chapter 20

The Health and Safety Officer was making his usual
nightly rounds, followed at a discreet distance by the
Finance Officer, just as when Dave had first seen them from
his study window. The first was planting official-looking
notices and the second was taking them down. On the
notices, in large red letters was printed the promise that any
visitor injured on the premises would be compensated in full
by the college authorities and the invitation to report all
such injuries to the Finance Officer without delay. The
Finance Officer was confiscating the notices and adding
them to the huge pile amassed since the return of the Safety
Officer after his spell in hospital.

This night, however, there was a difference. They
had both agreed to a cessation of hostilities at half-past ten
so that they could both smell gas in Dave's room and do
something about it. Neither had kept to the plan however.
The Health and Safety Officer had visited the room earlier
than arranged in order to effect a little malicious damage to
windows or light bulbs or mirrors which the Finance Officer
would have to make good. It was his usual practice to break
a window or two on his nightly rounds if for no other reason
than to make his tormentor pay up.

Unknown to him, the Finance Officer had also
visited the room before the agreed time and had turned on
the gas fire in order to make sure that they smelled the
agreed gas. So when they eventually met on the stairs at the
appointed hour and proceeded in frosty silence to the source

of the leak neither was prepared for the explosion that ensued.

"Do you smell gas in this room?" asked the Health and Safety Officer.

"I believe I do. Shall we investigate do you think?"

"I think we should. Will you turn on the light?"

"The switch does not seem to work. Or perhaps the light bulb is damaged. It is only what I would expect from that fellow Smith. Hang on a minute and I will strike a match."

Shortly afterwards he found himself at the bottom of the stairs and then on his way to hospital accompanied by his companion in crime.

One of the first on the scene was Mr Scott who had been nearby discussing with Mrs Erfert a plan to extricate Dave from his series of escalating disasters. They had just thought of something that might work when the two officers came flying past them. It was a plan that entailed utilising the same Academic Board that had been the source of the original trouble. The problem would be that the sensible party was usually outvoted by the Erfertian disciples. The odds had improved because the recent accident had reduced the loonies by at least one vote, or two if the two enemies continued their unholy alliance. Erfert would also vote for Dave.

Miriam Woodstock had never previously made a decision in her life and would probably not start now, except that she had been heard to shout for Dave's assassination at one stage. If the resignation specialist could be urged to resign it might help too. The news that the Finance Officer was to be released from hospital because his fall on top of the Health and Safety Officer had lessened his injuries both posed a problem and presented an opportunity to those wishing to manipulate the Board. The plan was to appeal to the sadistic nature of the Finance Officer. It must therefore involve the spending of money, but not too much money, and if possible, spent so as to provide something that the least number of people could enjoy. If the Finance man voted for it and the Religious Studies man voted against it on the grounds that the Science man had voted for it there was a chance that Mr Scott might just get his way. As the Finance man rather fancied himself with the ladies, Mrs Erfert agreed to work on him whilst he was still in need of a delicate hand to cool his fevered brow. Dave was also important to the plan and Mr Scott sent him a little note asking him to recall his civil servant's training to think up a mandarin's solution to a problem that had defied the Finance Officer for years. He also asked him to attend the next Academic Board and to play the game outlined by Mr Scott.

The Board came to order, or as near to order as the Board ever came. The Principal went on to matters arising from previous minutes. Since no decision had yet been taken on Dave's assassination or expulsion there was no minute to consider but one of the scientists raised it anyway.

"Principal, on behalf of my colleagues in the department I should like to move a resolution to the effect that we expel Mr David Smith."

"I should like to move an amendment to that," shouted the Amendment-In-Search-of-A-Resolution.

"And what might that be?" enquired the Principal.

"I should like to add the words; 'that bloody little sod,' before the name David Smith."

"And I should like to move an alternative amendment," said the Resignation Specialist.

"Yes," said the Principal.

"I should prefer the words 'bloody little swine' to 'bloody little sod'."

"Why is that?" enquired the Amendment-In-Search-Of-A-Resolution.

"Because it is more suitable," came the rejoinder.

"Nonsense," said the Amendment.

"Are you questioning my judgement?" the Resignation Specialist demanded.

"Doesn't everybody?" asked his adversary.

"I must ask you to withdraw that remark or I shall have to resign."

"Gentlemen," said Mr Scott soothingly. "Let us have a little more decorum if you please. We will never get anywhere in this way. I am of course very disappointed that Mr Lovatt has decided to resign but if that is what he wants that is what we must accept. May I, through you Mr Chairman, thank Mr Lovatt for all the hard work he has put in over the years and express the hope that he will feel able to join us again in the not too distant future? Thank you very much Mr Lovatt and good day to you." And so, before he knew what had hit him, Mr Lovatt was wheeled out of the room to the sound of a generous round of applause.

That was one less vote to worry about.

"Now let us get back to the resolution and the amendment," said Erfert.

"Before you do that can I say something?" asked Dave.

"No" roared everyone except Erfert and Scott.

"Yes, of course," said Erfert.

"I don't suppose it would make any difference if I apologised?" asked Dave hopefully.

"No," they all cried in unison.

"Yes, it would," replied the imperturbable Erfert.

"Could I just say that my own doctor and another specialist now agree with the other psychiatrist that I am no longer mad."

"Your own doctor does not know his business then," snapped the college quack. "And, if you are not insane it makes your behaviour all the more abominable."

"It's all my mother's fault," said Dave desperately trying to implement his doctor's advice. "She tried to smother me at birth, you know and I transferred her guilt to Dr Erfert. She tried again last night but she failed and I came to see that Dr Erfert was in no way to blame. So you see, now that I can see the full picture like the specialist experts do, I can admit to being mad and in doing so I become sane."

This ludicrous argument stuck in his throat but it appealed to quite a few of the resident crackpots who nodded their heads comprehendingly. It cut no ice, however with the huge abdomen of the scientist sitting next to him.

"First you are mad then you are not mad. Just what do you take us for?" he demanded. Dave did not dare tell him.

"It is a pity that your mother is so bad at smothering people," ventured another member, "She could have saved us all a lot of trouble."

"I do not know what to think I am sure," wailed Miriam Woodstock in her slightly contradictory fashion.

The Finance Officer said nothing but the Religious Studies man felt uneasy at being on the same side as the scientist with the abdomen and was seeing some merit in a seemingly miraculous conversion. He was about to declare his own change of mind when Mr Scott showed his mastery of this particular game.

"May I have the indulgence of the Board to introduce a new factor into the argument?" he asked at his oiliest best.

"Of course," agreed the Principal, "and what might that be?"

"The new swimming pool."

Even Erfert's appointees could see no obvious connection between a swimming pool and Dave's future but they were willing to be intrigued.

"What has that got to do with anything?" demanded the man whose forte was counting the chairs in lecture rooms to establish the room occupancy efficiency rate only to be outwitted by those members of staff who achieved one hundred per cent efficiency by the simple expedient of putting outside the room any chairs which were not occupied.

"I thought that we had no chance of a new swimming pool" said the man whose chief occupation was writing six page letters on the need to save paper and who himself saved paper by writing two three-page letters instead. "We have had it turned down three times by the D.E.S. to my knowledge."

"Precisely," said Mr Scott. "And so has the new Science Laboratory only this morning." He threw the letter of rejection on to the table in an effort to get the attention of the scientist's abdomen.

"Disgraceful," said the abdomen, "but I still don't see what this has got to do with the matter in hand."

"This young man's crime is that he came here to expose the Principal as a fraud and to show up the College," he patiently explained.

"There is some doubt about whether he is mad or not. Neither the Principal nor I think he is. Indeed the

Principal has offered to help him with his plan which is very generous of him I am sure. He is a little deranged perhaps but not mad in the ordinary sense of the word. No, his real crime is treachery. That is what the students with their commendable loyalty to the College hold against him."

"So he should be fired. Get to the point."

"Let us suppose that we could get the gamekeeper to turn poacher. Let us suppose that Mr David Smith undercover man from the D.E.S. could be turned, could become a double agent. Let us suppose that he could use his knowledge of the workings of the D.E.S. to get for us all those things that they have been refusing for years; your swimming pool, your science laboratory and your planetarium. The decision, surprisingly enough, was 'no' for the science department but 'yes' for a planetarium for the resident astrologer who writes the references."

His examples were well chosen to sway the votes in the game called Academic Board Manipulation. "He could do us far more good if we let him stay than all the attendant publicity that would arise if we threw him out."

"The idea of a double agent attracts me very much," said Erfert. "I knew quite a lot at Cambridge in the old days. I nearly joined the K.G.B. myself once but my wife was against it at the time."

Even Dave could see the mood changing and he realised that Mr Scott had left him an opportunity to jump in. "Well I can certainly help you to get your new swimming pool," he ventured. He now had the interest of the Board. He knew the problem well, as a matter of fact, because half the colleges in the country had had requests turned down by the

D.E.S. The Department always answered that there could be no money for an amenity that was for College use only, and as the Colleges did not want to share the pool with anyone else they did not pursue it. The D.E.S. insisted on a public pool within a private campus and the Finance Officer had a deep-rooted objection to large numbers of people enjoying themselves anyway. It would be bad enough if the students got some enjoyment out of it.

"If I may say so you played it wrong when you asked for a pool for College use only," he explained. "You were right to refuse to have it for public use but there is another category that you could have gone for. You should have asked for a pool for 'Community Use' and then define Community Use in a way that suits you best. It is obviously less that 'Public Use' and more than 'Private Use' but just what it is is anybody's guess. You can restrict the use of the pool to one-legged septuagenarians on a Tuesday afternoon between three and four o'clock if you want and it could still be termed 'Community Use'."

The Finance Officer loved it. A public pool that the public could not use appealed to his sadistic nature immediately. All he had to do now was to think of some reason for preventing the College from using it as well. Ideally a compliant Health and Safety Officer could shut it down or empty it of water but that was unlikely, to say the least. Others liked it too and a ripple of applause went round the room; the kind that had greeted his original disastrous hypnosis suggestion. But all that was in the past; Dave was now persona grata again.

"I support the suggestion," said the Finance Officer.

"And so do I," said the Abdomen.

"And I," shouted several others.

"And I agree too," said the Principal. "As you know, I have never believed that Mr Smith was mad. Indeed I am looking forward to helping him in his work against me. If we can put his expertise to work in other directions for the benefit of the College I would be only too delighted to make use of it. I understand that the police are no longer looking on him as a murderer, and a man answering the description of Arthur Pitts has been found in Warrington so the skeleton in the ladies toilets cannot be his. Can I suggest, therefore that we all look forward to working with Mr Smith instead of against him?"

Chapter 21

After the little matter of escaping charges of treason, insanity and murder, Dave felt like a rest and all the more so because the Principal was inundating him with more and more evidence of the Principal's shortcomings. He decided to spend a few days at home but his mother's tender care proved too much for him and he returned to College less than refreshed.

He was now something of a celebrity. A huge pile of letters awaited him at the porter's desk, most of them invitations to meet this or that lecturer to discuss 'matters of mutual interest' by which was meant a shopping list of items that they wanted to get from the D.E.S. The Finance Officer pestered him about how to stop more and more people from enjoying the new swimming pool which had now been approved in principle by the D.E.S. and the Science man was pestering him on how to get his new laboratory. So he was in no mood and no fit condition to help Erfert denounce himself as he seemed determined to do. Nevertheless, among his mail was a letter from the Principal asking him to come in and see him.

The Principal was in his room talking to a tall, athletic young man in sports jacket and slacks. The latter had taken advantage of an advertisement in the local paper inviting people with any problem to come and talk them over with Dr Erfert, who was of course a member of the Samaritans, the Citizen's Advice Bureau and the Community Health Council. It was all part of the policy of bringing together Town and Gown.

"Come in, Come in Mr Smith," said the Principal warmly. "You probably recognise Mr Young?" He did indeed recognise the centre forward of the local third division football team.

"To cut a long story short, Mr Young, my advice to you is that you consider suing the centre-back for assault and battery. In fact I reckon that you also have a good case against your own side's centre-back for preventing you from exercising your trade or profession."

"How do you work that out?" asked the footballer.

"Well you cost the club a half a million pounds in transfer fees didn't you?"

"Yes."

"And they bought you to score goals, didn't they?"

"Right"

"And you have not been scoring any?"

"Right again."

"Even though you scored them in profusion with your last club?"

"Correct."

"Well, I know you only came to see me to see if I could suggest ways of rolling over and diving to the ground after you have scored a goal to show your delight without having your own team injure you by diving on top, but it really will not come to that if you do not in fact score any goals. In the course of our conversation you seemed to imply that this was because you have been starved of passes by your colleagues in general and some of them in particular. I think you said that their remissness had in fact rendered you as sick as a parrot when at your last club you were always over the moon. It seems to me like restraint of trade in that starving you of passes renders you unable to carry out the job for which you were bought. It is something like secondary picketing and if it goes on your goals will dry up altogether and you will go down in the estimation of the crowd, drop in transfer value and be open to character assassination in the local press. I think it is a more serious matter than you originally thought."

"Gee thanks Doc. I had never thought of that. I was only bothered about getting a new spontaneous wiggle or pose when I scored. It never occurred to me that I was not scoring goals at all. Its great to talk to you about these things. Could you handle a court case for me if I sue?"

"Of course, my boy. I do a fair bit of court work these days. People come in here with all sorts of problems and I am usually able to show them that what they think is their problem is only a symptom of some deeper underlying malaise. You would be surprised how mistaken some people can be even about themselves."

"You can say that again," thought Dave, as the grateful but dim young man was shown out of the room. Erfert then turned to Dave.

"I asked you to come in this morning to see if I can be of any assistance in your project to denounce me. Perhaps this morning's counselling session has given you some ammunition?"

"Oh, no!" Dave assured him. "I have decided not to go ahead with that. Not after all the trouble you went to in defending me."

"Nonsense my boy. You must go ahead with it. What is the point of my defending you if you are not going to go ahead with such an interesting piece of research. I have already got together a lot of old diaries and things to help you and I am willing to explain anything that is not clear to you - that is unless you think that my own bias towards myself will vitiate the explanation, in which case I can explain to you the nature of my own self image, as a means of countering the flaws engendered by the self image in explaining the diaries, you understand."

Dave did not understand but he was too weary to argue as Erfert babbled on. "Unless you think that my wife would explain them better. She is of course not actually objective, being my wife, but her subjectivity is objective in the sense that she chose to marry me in the light of what she knew about me so what she has to say will have some validity if only to place my own subjective explanations in some sort of corrective or corroborative framework."

The only thing that Dave could think of saying was; "I should be very happy to take up your offer sir but as you know, my Teaching Practice begins next week and I will not have time to take up my project until I get it over with."

"Not to worry," Erfert assured him. "I will help you with that as well."

This was a double blow. Dave had already proved himself to be quite a poor teacher and with Erfert's help he looked like becoming a disastrous one. In normal circumstances Erfert was kept well away from students practising in the real world and no-one would thank Dave for giving him an entree into what was already for some a traumatic experience. Teaching Practice was a make-or-break time. Once in each of three terms the students were sent out to 'learn from Nellie' as one lecturer put it. Most managed to scrape through, especially if they were judged by the resident crew of Erfertians but the Final Teaching Practice was a crucial test of competence assessed by external examiners. They had to prepare and write up numerous lessons which would then be delivered not only to the class but also to visiting lecturers and class teachers and external examiners. A particularly nerve-wracking experience was waiting for the lists to go up telling the students which schools they were appointed to and to which lecturers they were allocated. Bob Forester proved to be unfortunate on both counts.

"Oh my God," he shouted. "I have drawn Auntie Mary." Auntie Mary was Mr Johnson, Art lecturer, mystic and part-time idiot. He was not so silly as to miss the various commissions that came his way which earned him hard cash outside college for work done inside it, but he was too silly to be looking after students in school. His great solution for all problems of classroom behaviour was 'to love them', 'them' being the little horrors who had started the problem in the first place.

If Bob Forester was disappointed, Martin Lockett was positively suicidal. Erfert had vaguely remembered that he had promised to tutor Dave Smith and had used his usual method of matching students to tutors by drawing names out of a hat. He remembered enough to put his own name in the hat but when the draw was made it came out alongside the name of Martin Lockett. When he saw the list, poor Martin could only stand there, stock still, mouthing feeble words which he could not quite force past his quivering lips. It was Bob who announced his dreadful fate to the others crowding round.

"He's drawn Herr Cutt," he shouted in amazement.

A hush descended upon the hitherto jostling crowd of eager young men and women. The whole bunch was stunned into immobility. Everyone knew that something terrible had happened. They all knew the score. They would all cover up all sorts of abnormalities at St. Brendan's. No-one was likely to do a Dave and spoil the game. But this was too much. The one unwritten rule that bound everyone together was that Erfert was never, repeat never, to be allowed near a real student in a real school situation. Dave dare not reveal any association with this cock up or his rehabilitation would have come to an instantaneous and painful end.

The unfortunate Martin Lockett was carried through the silent sympathetic crowd. He was rigid and cold with only the terror in his eyes to betray the slightest sign of life. His silent friends parted to allow his remains to be deposited in a corner seat near the bar where he stayed for a full three hours staring motionlessly at a succession of whiskies which well wishers deposited before him as non verbal tokens of their profound sympathy. And even when his pall bearers carried him off to his miserable attic room not one person spoiled the tribute by touching a single drop of his untouched martyr's drink.

It was three days before any sort of life returned to Martin Lockett and he was able to resume his promising career as an apprentice alcoholic. He presented himself at the Principal's door having fortified himself by finding and consuming his untouched drinks to be briefed about what was expected of him on the four-week Teaching Practice which was to follow.

"Come in. Sit down my boy. Come in. Sit down my boy," said the Principal. He was trying out one of his latest ideas which was to treat all interviews as if there was a third person present. He believed that the presence of a third person would make him that little bit more careful about how he treated people and how it would make for fairness and equality of treatment for all. From this basic idea he had progressed to actually addressing the third person and he was now very near to preferring the third person to most of the students that he encountered in the course of his duties. All this was however lost on the panic-stricken Martin Lockett who was white with fear, dizzy from lack of sleep and swaying from an excess of alcohol.

"Thank you sir," he stammered.

"I hope that you do not mind telling me all about yourself in front of a third party. Just say if you do and I will see you on my own."

Lockett's fuddled brain saw a chance of a way out.

"Frankly sir," he said "I do rather object to speaking in front of someone else. I think that Teaching Practice ought to be a very private affair between the two people most concerned."

"I see your point,"said Erfert. "Perhaps I ought to leave you two to sort it out."

"Or maybe you would want to hand me over to another tutor because of my impertinence."

"Nonsense, my boy. I shall do no such thing. What I will do is to give you my full and undivided attention with no distractions."

To Lockett's surprise the Principal said quite a few sensible things about how to prepare for the Practice by getting the appropriate notebooks, lesson plans and resources and it left him wondering if he had misjudged Erfert after all. Encouraged by what he had heard he made the fatal mistake of asking him a question. He explained that the primary school to which he had been attached had both vertical streaming and mixed ability teaching groups and he wanted to know how he was expected to cope not being used to either. He did not know that he had opened up Erfert's problem-solving technique which could be applied to any problem under the sun because it never actually produced any answers.

"That is a very good question, my boy." Rule number one of the technique was to praise the questioner. This would establish a relationship with him and also give one time to think. Rule number two was to repeat the question so as to be sure that it had been accurately posed.

"You have a class in which there is mixed ability teaching and vertical streaming. That is correct is it?"

By cleverly juxtaposing the terms of the question he had carefully gained more time and also clarified that this was indeed the same question. The next step was to clarify possible approaches to the answer.

"Now that we have established what the question really is let us analyse some possible approach strategies." Martin thought that sounded reasonable enough. But Erfert went on; "Suppose we start by looking at some of the things that we would obviously NOT do." This puzzled Martin but he went along with it nonetheless like a passenger who has missed his stop and stays on the bus in the hope that it will come round again.

"We would not dream of trying to answer the question without first defining our terms would we?" continued the Principal who then proceeded to take ten minutes to give various interpretations of the two terms used in the question, analysing each in accordance with the various sub-headings of his technique. When he had finished this task he returned to the mainstream argument,

"We would not attempt to solve such a question by doing nothing would we?" he asked, leaving Martin hoping against hope that they could do just that. "Therefore we must do something, n'est-ce-pas?" he proclaimed triumphantly. Martin just nodded.

"But in doing something we must critically assess the various effects that the different courses of action will have on the overall situation. If the effect of our action would be to change fundamentally the situation then we would have altered the original problem, wouldn't we? If that were the case we would no longer be solving the original problem and so the answer, although it might be effective, would not be relevant to the task in hand. By the very act of trying to solve the problem we have changed it so in that sense we have solved it but in another sense we have not. If it is no longer there to be solved then I suppose that we have solved it."

All this was too much for Lockett's fuddled brain and he was reduced to nodding dumbly throughout the discourse. Erfert seemed to be satisfied that he had solved something for he then brought it down to the class level by insisting that he would work on something for Martin, something scientific, something that would identify the children in each group. Martin hesitated to tell him that the register had already identified the children in each group and all he intended to do was to read it. In any event Erfert was unstoppable.

"We can perhaps work out a way of doing nothing in such a manner as to avoid our lack of action becoming a positive action in the sense of altering the original situation. If we can keep the status quo long enough to avoid altering the terms of the problem then we should be in a better position to solve it root and branch at a later date."

Martin was not quick enough to follow most of this and the Principal prattled on for some time until he suddenly went quite still and quiet, like a robot whose batteries had run out. Martin took advantage of the interlude, picked up his notes and quietly left the room to join his fellow students in the bar where they compared notes. From all the bits of advice that they had received they were able to put together some sensible points that would be of use on their impending Practice. It was a mark of their maturity that it was they rather than the majority of their tutors who could take the credit for their professional preparation.

Chapter 22

Dr Erfert was one of the few College Principals to be a member of both the Royal Historical Society and the Denis the Menace Fan Club at one and the same time. He took great delight in perusing the Beano to see if the editor had found space to include his latest letter and he was always happy to discover that his work found favour with the children of school age. He was therefore one of the few Principals who liked and was liked by children. They often called at his house to see if he was coming out to play. But on this particular morning he had to disappoint them for he was engaged on solving the problem that Martin Lockett had set him. Dave, on the other hand, was visiting his school for the first time and found the experience somewhat daunting. Schools treated students with varying degrees of kindness. Dave and his female student colleague were ushered into a very small room which served as the head's study, the staff room, the sick-bay and the store room. It was a tiny room to begin with; found in one corner of an old 'Board School' of the type the D.E.S. consistently maintained no longer existed. The school was built around a central hall and all the classrooms ranged round the central hall-cum-gym. There were at most a half a dozen staff in the school but when they all crowded into this one room there was literally no room to turn round. If yard duty had been invented for no other reason than to relieve the congestion in that room it would have been well worth it. With two students and a visiting tutor also shoe-horned in it resembled the Black Hole of Calcutta or a Japanese tube train in the rush hour. It was the task of the teacher on yard duty to close the door on the struggling mass inside and push in any protruding body parts. It was also her duty to release them at the end of the break.

Even so Dave thought himself lucky not to have drawn one of the bright modern schools designed by the specialist eccentrics of the D.E.S.'s Architectural Branch. Students in gleaming modern buildings usually had truncated Practices because the buildings were more often than not closed for repairs to the fabric, the flat roofs or the High Alumina Cement concrete beams. If it was not repairs to the fabric it was the failure of the central heating systems that caused the problems. Teachers would refuse to teach in icy conditions, caretakers would refuse to mend the boilers because it was not their job, manufacturers would refuse to honour guarantees if anyone else had touched the boilers and invariably only arrived in school holiday time to inspect faulty equipment. Often enough the problem was solved by bussing the children back to the old 'Board School' from which they had recently been liberated. The students in these schools had a relatively easy time of it being frequently sent back to college. Some of them even got days off for the ceremony in which the architect received a certificate of merit for his great new showpiece. The only thing to stop such ceremonies was when the caretakers, prompted by their unions, refused to open up the schools. As only they could do so, there was a stand-off particularly if disgruntled staff refused to pass the picket line of one man. Then they could stretch out the dispute indefinitely.

But if all else failed the students in all schools had to face up to the daunting task of actually teaching real children. Whatever art they employed in this task was learned from the teachers in the school rather than from the staff of the college, particularly Erfert's hand-picked team. Not all the staff of the schools were beyond reproach of course. The head teacher of Jane's school paused in his introduction and welcome to the school to explain the progressive methods employed there and to belt two boys round the ears for not sitting up straight for the visitors. Some schools were in fact run by secretaries whilst the heads got on with more important things such as tending the greenhouse. There was one school which was competently run by the head teacher's wife, a formidable lady of ample proportions but with no corresponding educational qualifications. And there were those delightful schools run by dedicated men and women whose career coincided with their vocation and whose efforts made their little worlds into places of enlightenment, peace and order.

If only Dave could have found such a haven he would have been happier than he was. He had struck lucky with his tutor because of Erfert's mistake; it was too much to hope that he should also have struck lucky with his school. It turned out that the junior school to which he was assigned was in a rough area and had more than fifty per cent of its pupils from families of various ethnic groups recently arrived in the town. The children and the ethnicity of the intake did not cause any problems other than the need for some remedial English lessons and cultural understanding. The pupils were beautiful, smiling, well-behaved little creatures who were bright and willing to learn but the head had something of a problem. He reacted to the most innocent of opening remarks in a way that surprised Dave on the very first day.

"I see that you have a large number of coloured children," remarked Dave for want of something to say.

"Yes," said the head very sharply, "but they are black, not coloured."

"That must be a problem," Dave innocently observed.

"Problem ? Who said that we have a problem?" he almost snarled. "We have no problem here, no problem at all. We have never had a problem at all here. Ask the teachers. They will tell you that we have no problem, no problem at all." And with that he left the scene still muttering that he had no problem. It was left to one of the staff to explain to Dave what the real problem was.

It seemed that the school had been a perfectly normal educational institution until the influx of immigrants some years before. They themselves posed no problem but, once their presence was known, the school had been besieged by sociologists with their notebooks and tape recorders demanding to be shown the problem so that they could suggest solutions. It was in vain that the head tried to assure them of his complete lack of any racial problem. Solutions they had aplenty so there must have been a corresponding problem. Letters of sympathy arrived by every post. The unions demanded special concessions from the Local Authority. Advisers were sent down to give specialist help. Questionnaires from well-meaning busybodies littered the head's desk like confetti. White parents appeared in delegations. The head was very nearly ready to admit that he had a problem in order to get a bit of peace.

Dave's arrival did not help much either because being less intelligent than some, he began bending over backwards to avoid any trouble over racial issues. He struggled to find more acceptable ways of referring to the children other than 'coloured' or 'black' or 'Asian' and his predicament spread to his lessons. In a lesson on Red Indians he tried referring to ' indigenous inhabitants of North America' but the children were quite uncomprehending. When he distributed paper and crayons to draw these indigenous peoples his conscience told him that some neutral colour other than red should be used. It was a misconceived performance worthy of Erfert himself and it came very near to giving the school a problem that various 'experts' confidently assumed it had.

He wasn't a very good teacher anyway and he struggled desperately to keep control over his lessons. He could see that his tutor was not too happy with his performance and he knew only too well that it would be terrible to be failed at this stage of his career and qualification was all important if only to give some credence to his criticisms of the system at St. Brendan's. His northern common sense told him that he ought to seek help from the staff and from his tutors in the various subject areas but when he asked the P.E. man for help he received the somewhat unhelpful advice to; "run 'em round the field until they bloody drop." The geography teacher was more helpful. She advised him to try to interest them and suggested that he capture the imagination by bringing in something like a volcano that gave off real smoke. When Erfert heard of this he promptly invented the chemical formula for one but it worked so well that on lighting it, Dave had to evacuate the room as clouds of smoke and sparks took over the class.

Dave had to face it: he was just not cut out for teaching. His limited intellectual pretensions made him a rather unimaginative practitioner. At Creative Writing he tried his best but he was not really up to it. He was not helped by coming up against a deadly honest child.

"Now I want you all the close your eyes," he said in his most gentle if patronising voice. They not only understood what he wanted but they performed the task with speed and enjoyment.

"Now can you all see the farmyard?" he asked. They all nodded.

"Can you see the chickens?" They all nodded vigorously.

"Can you see the geese?" This time they all nodded vigorously except for one little girl who insisted with a worried look on her face that she could not in all honesty see the geese in question.

"Of course you can," he coaxed.

"I can't sir," she claimed.

"You can," he said, much more sternly.

"I can't sir," she insisted with tears in her eyes and a sob in her voice.

Dave was getting more and more out of his depth. Not only was he unused to dealing with crying little girls but he had no idea of how to depart from his set prepared routine. So he went back to his more gentle style and took her back over the mental picture that he had established so far. He ascertained that they were agreed that she could see the chickens and the farmyard.

"Now look carefully over there near the chickens. There is a gate and the geese are near the gate. Can you see the gate?"

"Yes, sir," she answered to his great relief but the rest of the class, annoyed at the introduction of something that they had not seen simply roared; "No."

"Oh yes you can," Dave roared back.

"Sir," said one little boy, "the geese that I saw were not near a gate; they were near a pond."

"That's not fair," complained another. "You never told us there was a pond."

"I can't see the pond either," said the first little girl.

"Ok, Ok," said Dave. "We'll try something else. Look let us pretend that we are up in an aeroplane and we are looking down at the scene below. Now what might we see down there?"

"Fields, sir."

"Good. Anything else?"

"Animals, sir."

"Yes, and ...."

"Buildings, sir."

"Good ... and ..."

His tutor, Mrs Sudden, stirred uneasily at the back of the classroom somewhat alarmed at the prospect of seeing a creative writing lesson that was going nowhere fast. Dave's contribution seemed to be to say "yes, and ..." to every suggestion made. But at least he had overcome the problem of the missing geese. She sidled up to the front of the class and whispered in his ear; "Don't just say 'yes' every time someone gives you a name. Take up the answer and add to it, embroider it. Make it more interesting. Add a word or two to increase their vocabulary. If they say 'fields' say to them; what kind of fields? Are they beautiful green fields?"

"Right," said Dave, who was by now completely demoralised by his failure to make contact with the children or with the subject matter. All he was waiting for, like the novice boxer that he was, was to hear the bell which would herald the end of a disastrous round one.

"Jimmy, tell me again what you would see from the aeroplane."

"Fields, sir," came the prompt reply.

"Good lad, Jimmy but don't just say 'fields.' Say 'beautiful green fields or something like that'. Embroider it a little."

Mrs Sudden quietly left the room before she had a fit. She did not see how Dave could pass his qualifying examination and she did not want to face him with her verdict after so short an acquaintance. The difficulty was that if she recommended that he receive specialist help from one of her colleagues he was likely to get a lot worse. The specialist in creative writing, one Donald Whitgift, was one of Erfert's appointees and if anyone was put on this earth in order to show students how not to teach a creative writing lesson it was he. Still she had to do something so she made an appointment for Dave to see him.

Whitgift was delighted to help. He informed him that he was not surprised that he was having difficulty because he was a pretty colourless sort of chap quite unlike himself who was dynamic and charismatic. The solution was to make the lesson interesting and he would come along to demonstrate how to do it. He duly arrived on the appointed day and informed the class that; "Today we are going to do something exciting." Getting nowhere with the opening gambit he went on to ask; "Who can tell me some exciting jobs that people do?"

"Sir, a Spaceman," shouted one helpful soul, but he did not impress Whitgift who just turned on him with a terrible look of scorn and sneered, "And just how many astronauts do you know then? You can count on the fingers of one hand the number of people who are ever going to get to the moon. Try to be a bit more realistic."

"Sir, a Secret Agent like James Bond," tried another youth.

"The lives of these secret agents are not as exciting as they are made out to be in the films you know," he said with a pained expression on his face. "Most of it is just routine."

With that the class gave up trying to help him and just sat back waiting for some sort of mighty revelation that would inevitably follow. Nothing could have been more disappointing. His exciting job turned out to be some out of

the way occurrence that might appear to a postman on his daily rounds or some mishap to a window cleaner . He even qualified these epic stories by telling them that the number of accidents per thousand window cleaners was remarkably small so the mishap described would be out of the ordinary. Lest they ran away with the idea that they could write what they wanted to, Whitgift then proceeded to dictate the opening paragraph of the story that was to be creatively written and to supply them with a list of words that he judged suitable to the task in hand. It was, as he explained in a loud whisper to Dave, "to keep the little monkeys straight and direct their creative impulses along acceptable lines. Of course it is only my opinion, but it is the right one."
He would have gone on with this helpful demonstration if one bold little girl had not raised her hand and asked; "Please sir can we have Mr Smith back to teach us again?" Whitgift took this as an enormous compliment to himself and proudly handed the class back to Dave saying that he had saved the situation and they were now ready for him again and he was not to spoil it. He had helped Dave in fact for the latter now realised that there were worse teachers in the world than himself and he threw himself into the rest of the Practice with renewed zest if not much skill.

He even allowed himself to be tutored by Miriam Woodstock, another of Erfert's appointees and a joke among her colleagues for never being able to make up her mind. They mimicked her with such renderings as: "Well that is my opinion and if you don't like it I will change it." She could not make up her mind about how indecisive he was but others could write a book about it. Students seeking help just could not get an answer out of her. They had to stalk her through the college because she had numerous ways of avoiding people.

Dave experienced her non-tuition at close quarters when he asked her whether he should use block capitals or lower case letters when writing on the board for eight year olds to read.

"Do what you think best in the circumstances," she replied.

"Is one more favoured than the other?"

"Both have a part to play"

"Could you tell me what kind of part they each play?"

"Quite a large part."

"Are there any dangers in using one or the other?"

"Of course."

"What should I avoid then?"

"I should avoid some of the more harmful effects."

"Could you give me an example?"

"That would depend upon the circumstances."

He gave up that particular quest quite soon but he was not to know that Miss Woodstock's style was also doing him down with the head teacher.

"He is a nice lad," said the head to her about Dave.

"Yes, indeed he is,"she agreed.

"Solid and reliable."

"Yes, I am sure he is."

"Although he makes some mistakes that experience will put right."

"I do not think that he is perfect""

"What kind of mark are you thinking of giving him?" he asked.

"What do you think he should get?" she countered.

"I am not sure what the pass mark is."

"It varies."

"How does he compare with your other students?"

"I have seen three others so far and he is not unlike them."

"Is he better or worse?"

"That depends on what criterion you use."

"And what criterion do you use?"

"Me? I always go by the book."

"And what sort of order would you put the four students in?"

"I think that they fit the normal curve of distribution."

"Can you do that with only four students?"

"No. But I also use my judgement and invariably I find myself in agreement with the Head's judgement so I think that that bears out that my method is pretty accurate."

At which point the head gave up.

Dave was not to know it but his path was to cross hers on more than one occasion outside the formal situation. One night, feeling particularly dispirited over his lack of class room success he turned to his faithful C.B. radio for some solace and had an interesting conversation with Batman and Robin who seemed to be a father and son combination. Then he tuned into Delilah's wavelength and found her sultry, smooth seductive voice something of a calming influence on his frayed nerves

"One four for a copy," he began.

"Hello, is that you Caveman?" whispered the sultry siren. "How are you you naughty boy? It is ages since I have spoken to you. I have missed you you know."

"I am sorry that I have not been in touch Delilah but I have been very busy."
"I wonder if I can guess what has been keeping you busy?" she answered slyly and suggestively.

"Oh its just that things have been getting on top of me lately and people who are supposed to help me are not doing so. To be honest I am just fed up."

"You poor boy you are in need of a little gentleness from Delilah. Why don't we meet so that I can soothe your fevered brow?"

"OK," he said with a sigh. "Where shall we meet?"

"Do you know the main gate of St. Brendan's College?"

"Yes," he said, getting the wind up at the prospect of Delilah being one of the students.

"I will meet you at the front gate in half an hour. Don't keep Delilah waiting."

He put the microphone of his Amstrad 901 rig back on his hook at the same instant as Delilah switched off her Rotel rig and rushed away to the bathroom to transform herself into as near an imitation of Marta Hari as it was possible for Miriam Woodstock to become in half an hour. Indecision was a thing of the past when she was on her rig. She could play out all her fantasies to her heart's content. But once off it she had no stomach for the action. So as the two of them approached the porter's lodge, Dave walked straight past as if on his way out and Miriam asked the porter if there was any mail for her as she was expecting an important letter.

Chapter 23

The mandarin, his minion and his cat were in conference. Important decisions had to be made. The Secretary of State was to visit the north on a major tour of educational institutions and a new policy had to be produced in time for her to announce it. It would be truer to say that existing policy had to be dressed up to look as if it were new and dynamic. Her white paper on Expanding the System had heralded the biggest contraction of the Service ever so now it was time to expand again. But the slogan was clapped out and no alternative was suggesting itself, certainly not one that seemed to save money, commend multiculturalism and encourage feminism.

"What we need is something that nobody can argue with. Something like we got away with when we centralised under our control all the opt-out schools and did it under the banner of decentralisation and parental choice. Nobody could possibly argue against parental choice even if we never granted any."

"Yes that was brilliant,"agreed his minion wistfully. "It was even better when we gave them a bribe to opt out and then cut back the funds of everyone else to pay for it."

"And don't forget that we then cut back on the funds of the opt-out schools as well," cried the mandarin gleefully.

"Ideas like that don't come up very often though," mourned the minion. " Unless ..."

"Unless what?" demanded his boss impatiently.
"Unless we can get Dr Erfert to help us again."

"Of course, get him on the phone will you Peter?"

"Dr Erfert, hello, how are you? I just thought that I would give you a ring to thank you for your suggestion about changing the name of the D.E.S. again. Your idea gives just the right sort of message to the outside world. It looks as though we have had a major reorganisation here... er, which of course we have had...." He realised that he was letting the cat out of the bag at this point so he hurriedly got on to the real business in hand.

"By the way, I was wondering if you could give a little attention to a further problem that we have at the moment. As you may know, we have stopped closing colleges and are now minded to adopt an expansionist mode. In fact we wish to take in record numbers of students over the next ten years. Unfortunately there is no money in the kitty to pay for it and we are getting some flak from the backwoodsmen in the system who claim that students are suffering. I think it originated with some students who reckoned that they had no beds to sleep on for the first three weeks of term because of overcrowding in their colleges. Even when we went out of our way to find them beds in Salvation Army Hostels they just turned their complaints against libraries and lack of resources. They will be on about food next. There really is no pleasing them so we ignore them. But with the Secretary of State having to make a major policy speech when she visits such institutions we have to be careful not to exacerbate the situation. Ideally, we would like her to announce some big initiative, one that enables us to expand, spend no money and still be capable of being defended at the despatch box as being enlightened. Can you think up anything on those lines?"

"Certainly," said Dr Erfert, who was never fazed by anything. He did not appreciate the Machiavellian undertones but was only too willing to help a friend in need. "As a matter of fact what you say fits in very nicely with what I am working on at the moment."

"And what is that?"

"Quality," said the Doctor.

"Quality?" echoed the mandarin puzzled by what even he would concede sounded like a contradiction in terms.

"And cost effectiveness," added Erfert.

Now he was talking! The mandarin gripped the phone in excitement at the brilliance of the man who could link quality with saving money. Who could possibly argue with a speech that demanded a quality service that was value for money? He could see the headlines now. In fact he usually issued the desired headlines with his press releases anyway and tired or lazy journalists were only too happy to accept them. His knighthood would be assured and he would become as famous as his revered predecessor who had introduced the system of Payment By Results in the middle of the nineteenth century.

"Tell me more," he begged.

Erfert was oblivious to the mandarin's real intentions but was by now happily working out details of his idea. He had several carefully graded items that made up quality. There was Quality Assurance, Quality Control, Quality Audit, Quality Validation and Quality Accreditation for starters. All this was lost on the civil servant until Erfert suddenly said, "And Quis custodies ipsos custodiet?"

"That is very interesting," said the mandarin, whose public school education had not been wasted. It enabled him to recognise Latin even if he could not translate it. What it turned out to mean was to prove a God-send to him. Who was to ensure and inspect the quality of institutions and who was to ensure the quality of the inspectors? This could provide him with a means of controlling a quality that he himself could define and an army of inspectors who not only inspected but inspected each other ad infinitum. Not only that but cost-effectiveness could be quality. The cheaper the better. It was perfect. Erfert was a genius. He deserved a medal. He would be in the New Year's Honours Lists without a doubt.

"There is just one thing," he put to Erfert. "How do I explain that doubling the number of students in say your college, with no increase in staff, and perhaps a cut in resources, actually improves quality?"

"Simple," said Erfert. "We devise new teaching methods that are up-to-date, vital and student centred."

"Such as?"

"Well it might differ with the different subjects, of course, but take what used to be called History for instance. The method of lecturing to thirty students is no different for forty, is it? or fifty? In this technological age all you need is a link up and you do not even need the lecture hall."

"But what about tutorials?"

"Yes. What about tutorials? Six people in a room with a lecturer is rather wasteful of resources, isn't it? Six people in a room without a lecturer, but student-led is much better; student-run tutorials are much more participative and more economical to boot. Students are quite capable of marking their own essays and marking other students' essays too. The lecturer's time would be much better spent on training them how to teach each other."

As he prattled on he was oblivious to the fact that he was presenting the D.E.S with a ready made plan for wrecking the whole of the educational system of the country. His fellow principals would have wrung his neck if they had known. The mandarin thanked him, used him, and forgot him, preferring to take the credit for what was going into the forthcoming speech himself.

Erfert meanwhile, settled back to read the Beano. The leading member of the Dennis the Menace Fan Club then gave his attention to helping Martin Lockett solve his little problem with the same generosity that he had bestowed on the mighty civil servant.

Eventually he had satisfied himself on the matter and took himself off to the school where Martin was just about to start a lesson. He informed the student that he had indeed come up with a way of testing the age and ability ranges of children in vertically streamed classes.

Pausing only to chat to the delighted children about Desperate Dan's Cow Pie Suppers, he proceeded to take over the lesson and to distribute various sheets of coloured paper on which were printed passages about the English Civil War and some questions for the children to answer. The actual distribution caused a good deal of chaos in the class because he sent some round from the front some from the middle and some from the back. In order to reduce some of the confusion he was reduced to shouting out the colours of the paper that each should have received, only to be confounded by one little girl who shouted back that she was colour-blind and could make no sense of his instructions. He noted down her name as a suitable subject for a future research topic and sorted out her papers for her. He then asked the class to read the passages and to answer the questions.

One of the questions asked the children to "Write down any of the words that you do not understand" and this the children duly did. Then Martin collected the papers while Erfert entertained the class with THE LATEST ADVENTURES OF KORKY THE CAT which he read from an advance copy of the comic that he had received for review purposes. Erfert then left the school to "refine his raw data" and to "correlate the results". Had the children known what he was about they would have been interested to see how his conclusions matched up with their own unerring knack of placing almost everyone in the class in order of cleverness.

As it happened Erfert's conclusions matched up with nothing at all but, because he was who he was, they caused an awful stir in local educational circles. It turned out that all the known bright children ended up at the bottom of the class and all the duffers were at the top. In vain did Martin and the class teacher try to point this out to Erfert. In vain did they try to fathom out why the results were so wrong. It was the children, in the end who gave them the clue. It seems that all the bright children had been bright enough to read the passage and bright enough to realise that they did not understand some of the words. The less able ones had stumbled over the passage and had not been bright enough to know that they did not understand some of the words. For one reason or another, not least the physical task of writing them down, the less able children had fewer words on their lists and came out top in the scores. It was a juvenile case of Erfert's theory of enlarged, or expanded, ignorance.

If it had stopped there all would have been well. But when the results had been fed through Erfert's mini-computer and when the local Education Authority took an interest in what the great man was doing and when parents got wind of it, instead of being dismissed as the rubbish they were, the results became something of a cause celebre.

Erfert could not be wrong so a public enquiry was called for to see why so many children had been wrongly placed in the past. Victimisation was suspected, resignations called for. Parents were prepared to engage legal opinion to fight for their children's rights. Erfert was in great demand to show how scientific results were far superior to subjective opinions be they those of teachers or parents. Any teacher who questioned the results was obviously guilty of a cover-up, certainly incompetent and probably a subversive. It was all the more distressing to the chairman of the local education committee because the area was shortly to be visited by the Secretary of State and the word was that quality was the thing to be achieved. It was eventually solved by Erfert's suggestion that the local quality control had shown up deficiencies in the quality of delivery and that these defects had now been put right. The one quality outweighed the other so all was well.

Chapter 24

The Welsh are a funny lot and St. Brendan's had more than its fair share of them because of an old boy who, having achieved the impossible by getting a job in a closed Welsh community, insisted upon sending his old boys to his old college. Some of them were more trouble than they were worth but they were tolerated because of the contribution they undoubtedly made to the rugby team, the Gilbert and Sullivan Society and the choir. Alun Evans had no such saving graces and he occupied the room next to Dave.

When Dave learned that the Secretary of State was to visit the school to which Evans was attached it gave him the idea that Evans could fire some of his bullets for him. He did not hold out much hope that the Secretary of State was any better than others he had encountered but it was at least worth a try. So he worked hard on Evans only to discover that he was wasting his time. Evans needed no lessons from Dave about how to annoy English Secretaries of State. He was still smarting from his interview with Mr Scott who had described his last lesson as the inappropriate putting over the irrelevant.

"I don't really see how you make that out," he had stormed at the Vice Principal, who had calmly replied that he did not think that parents on a Lancashire housing estate sent their offspring to school to learn how to count up to ten in Welsh.

"I think that they would be all the better for it," answered the fervent Welsh nationalist and he thereby won the argument because like all arguments about curriculum theory, it was won by the vehemence with which the protagonist insists on his right to teach exactly what he wishes.

It was only to be expected that he carried his vehemence and his Welsh nationalism to extraordinary lengths on the day of the VIPs' visit. As was usual on such visits, she had a strict timetable to adhere to and one which allowed for only a whistle-stop tour of the tumble-down school where he was currently practising his black arts.

But those few minutes were of very great importance to the assembled local dignitaries who ranged from the Mayor to the lady Chairman of Governors, local councillors and officials and the police chief of the area. There was a faint hope of getting a new school out of the visit if only she proved sensitive to local pressure.

She arrived a little late, "all flashing teeth and hair-do,"as one local resident declared. She dispensed grace and charm all around as she went on a tour of the classrooms; until she arrived at the room where Alun Evans was observing a lesson given by his class teacher. Evans was dressed in denims with patches sewn inexpertly on the elbows and knees. He could have been a destitute window cleaner. His long hair fell over his shoulders in a way which tended to disguise his sex - which was Welsh. So was his height, his weight, his brain and his poetic soul. Everything about him was Welsh. He was a living, breathing Welsh socialist of the old school.

The elegant lady entered his room and asked a few pleasant questions of the children before addressing the window cleaner at the back. She asked him who he was and on hearing through the grunts and snorts that he was a student, she asked him about his course and about its quality. Without removing his bottom from his seat, the long-haired yobbo answered in a series of grunts.

"And do you like it here?" she persevered.

"Not much," was the only reply she received.

"May I ask why?" she said.

"No," came the curt reply.

By way of further explanation he went on to explain that someone born with an English silver spoon in her mouth could not be expected to understand the feelings of ordinary working class people and especially those of oppressed colonial minorities and students. He then launched into a bitter attack on the government's policy towards schools, higher education, students, grants and in particular the luring of thousands of young teachers straight to the scrap heap of unemployment.

It was a tribute to her political stature that she took all this without flinching but she still ought to have known better than to try to argue with a Welshman. Well used to defending the indefensible and vacillating policies of her department she tried every trick in the book. She tried patronising him and then her tremendously sincere and sympathetic approach. She tried platitudes that were treated with rude guffaws and ruder gestures. She tried rhetorical questions but he insisted upon answering them. She tried her famous stare-them-straight-in-the-eye look but found it difficult to match the stare of the two malevolent orbs that were half-hidden by the mass of greasy hair.

All this took up precious minutes. The scheduled time for departure came and went and the official party shuffled uneasily. The Chief Education Officer muttered that someone ought to separate these two before the whole day was ruined. The head teacher politely moved in to call time but neither heeded him. The VIP was a seasoned campaigner who had by now slipped into automatic pilot. And so it went on. Frantic phone calls flashed to and fro between school and the Education Offices to rearrange the whole programme. In the end the Secretary of State had to be half dragged away, still shouting after her bits of her party's election manifesto. Evans just sat there impervious to the shambles around him and convinced that the whole episode had proved him right anyway.

Nothing much happened until the V.I.P had been seen off the premises, still shouting out of the open window of the car as it sped away. Then the fireworks began. Mrs Alice Carter O.B.E, Chairman of Governors sent for the Head. The Head sent for the lad. The lad sent for his tutor. The tutor asked the Principal for his advice. The lad was sent packing from the school partly because of what he had done and partly for his own safety because Mrs Carter had her string of expensive pearls in her hands and was threatening to strangle him with them. Her fury was mainly due to the fact that she had had no chance to stress the needs of her dilapidated school to the important visitor.

All this presented a ticklish problem for the college. An apology seemed to be in order but some of the staff were showing distinct signs of sympathy with the young man.

They thought that it was great that one so young should stand up for his principles no matter what those principles were. Tory members of staff might think it outrageous that a member of the government should be treated in that way by a hooligan in denims but the few Welsh members tried to raise it at Academic Board as an unprovoked attack on a defenceless Welsh country boy, an innocent stranger in a foreign country, by a representative of organised capitalism.

It was up to the Principal to sort it out and Mr Scott cringed at what he might come up with. The school repeatedly claimed that the Secretary of State had been outraged by her treatment and had left the school in disgust. The lad claimed that this was only true in the sense that it was entirely accurate but in no other sense. Moreover she had given as good as she got and had been half responsible for the debacle.Dr Erfert inevitably put his finger on the weak point in the Opposition's argument. He shrewdly suspected that the lady in question was sufficiently battle hardened not to send in complaints herself. Most of the twenty four received had come from the school itself. They all claimed however that she had been outraged by her treatment. Erfert decided that he had to visit the school. On his arrival he corrected a few spelling mistakes on the official notice-board and with this piece of one-upmanship under his belt, proceeded to address the aggrieved audience.First of all he explained how unhappy the college was about the whole sad affair and then he explained that as he would be seeing the Secretary of State next week he would personally explain how much it was regretted. This made them stir uneasily for they had been unrestrained in their description of her outraged feelings and had not bargained on anyone actually checking out these things with her. But his next statement took them completely by surprise.

"I shall have to check with her that she does not mind the full page advertisement in the Daily Mirror, of course."

"The WHAT?" exclaimed the Chairman of the Governors.

"We feel so strongly about it that we are taking out a full page advertisement in the Daily Mirror so that our apology will be as public as possible. But I must make sure that she would not find it politically inexpedient."

By this time they were squirming on their seats. They had no desire to see their school on the pages of the national press and they had no wish to see their extravagant claims put to the test. They decided to assure him that the incident had not really been all that bad after all. The boy had certainly been impetuous but certainly not outrageous. Erfert however insisted on going on with his plan and it needed a letter from the D.E.S. itself to put him off his stroke. The D.E.S. had no intention of letting the Daily Mirror loose on a headline that inevitably would read like a young student's nightmare of having been sacked from a school simply for daring to advance a differing view from that of the Secretary of State. For one reason or another the incident passed into history. In fact it went further than into history. It had never existed at all. Whether Erfert knew he was being clever in all this is open to doubt but he had once more successfully employed rules of the game to the benefit of St. Brendan's.

Chapter 25

The Under-Secretary of State was feeling more than usually exhausted. He and his aide had spent the whole morning supervising a team of three underlings who were desperately trying to locate Preston on a map. When they eventually found it and confirmed that it was north of the Mersey they immediately lost interest in it and turned to other business. Anything north of the Mersey should in their opinion, be turned over to the Colonial Office anyway.

It was at this point that Theophilus pushed a sardine-flavoured envelope across the table. It contained Dr Erfert's proposals for a full page advertisement in the Daily Mirror.

The instinct for self preservation caused the mandarin to know at once that the advertisement would never see the light of day so he ordered replies to be sent to those who had complained which played down the whole issue.

"What kind of reply shall I send them," asked his aide.

"Oh the usual kind of standard letter which makes it look as if it is a personal one to each recipient. Thank them for bringing it to our attention. Tell them that it is being investigated and that they can take it for granted that we will act when necessary."

"And will we?"

"Don't be silly."

He then went on to read the rest of Dr Erfert's letter. It congratulated him on the brilliant plan to send an undercover man to St. Brendan's in order to spy on him and how happy he was to help the boy with the investigation.

"What a great man he is." said the mandarin. Then he asked his aide what all this was about a spy.

"Did we really do that?" he asked.

"I believe we did," came the reply.

"Who is this Dave Smith fellow and are we paying him?"

"He is that subversive fellow who used to work here and we got rid of him because he was not sound. He has obviously been stirring up trouble for Dr Erfert. There is some talk that he is mad."

"I cannot say that I remember him unless he was that northern fellow who insisted on importing text books from Somalia to make up a supposed deficiency in our school libraries."

"No that was another one. We got rid of him."

"Well get rid of this one as well. We are certainly not paying anyone to be a nuisance to Dr Erfert when he has helped us a good deal in the past. Put him on the sick list.

Give him a pension. We do still have break-down pensions don't we?"

"We have the pensions all right but we have no funds in the kitty. They were all used up by a horde of disenchanted head teachers who applied by the hundred when they were first announced."

"I have noticed how delicate head teachers seem to be these days. Anyway find a way of getting rid of Smith or whatever his name is. What about failing him on teaching practice? Then declaring that anyone who fails teaching practice cannot in all conscience be employed at the D.E.S. dealing with schools where you have to have some sort of credibility."

"I doubt if Dr Erfert would play ball with that one. He seems to like the fellow. But as teaching practice is in the hands of external examiners rather than the college it should be relatively simple to find an inspector to do the job for us."

"OK. Do it."

"And if the inspector will not play ball?"

"You have been reading too many books that tell you that the members of Her Majesty's Inspectorate are proud of their independence, an independence which is based upon receiving a personal commission from the Queen."

"Well, aren't they?"

"Not any more. Don't you remember that we threatened to privatise the lot of them and now they are falling over themselves to do what we want?"

"Oh yes, of course. Shall we get Dickie Biggs-Humphries? He is sound enough."

"No try that archaeologist woman whom we appointed er ... I mean Her Majesty appointed ... when she unfortunately lost her job in a college which we closed down last year."

"Mabel Croxteth. Well we could of course but you do remember that it was because of her that we closed down the college in the first place?"

"Not to worry. Just get on with it. But let her get her instructions from some intermediary. I don't care how she does it or what else she does. But get Dave Smith failed."

As a matter of fact he was worrying needlessly. Dave Smith was doing most of the work for him. He was not a very good teacher and he was not getting very much help from Erfert's appointees.

Before the students could qualify for the profession they had to spend several weeks in school on a final teaching practice and they had to endure the ordeal of a visit from an external examiner. The culmination of the whole process was a grand meeting of all lecturers and all external examiners to decide who should pass and who should fail. This meeting was a kind of war-game. It had its own rules and set-piece moves. A preliminary skirmish took place earlier in the week when the college did its very best to render the external examiners as drunk as possible and to keep them that way. It was not always easy for even a bad student to get himself failed.

The rules of the game meant that the script of the meeting could be predicted. It never varied. The external examiner would have an opening gambit; something like;

"Well I have seen Mr Monks teaching the ten year olds and quite frankly I do not feel as if I can pass him."

This was the cue for his tutor to express hurt surprise and to express the opinion that the boy was worth at least a "B" grade.

"I certainly did not see a "B" quality in the lesson he delivered today," was the obvious reply from the external examiner.

"Yes but the lesson you saw today was not a representative one. I have seen him six times and you have only seen him the once. Everything I saw was of a "B" quality so you must have caught him on an off day."

"I may have seen him only once but I have seen six other students and I can compare him with them and he is not a "B" quality student. In fact he was worth less than a student to whom I have awarded a "C" mark."

"I hope you have borne in mind that the children had just come back from the baths and that they were in no mood for a lesson on fractions and that the student was suffering from a very bad cold contracted by standing bare-headed at the graveside of his best friend who died in tragic circumstances only last week?"

"I understand all that but I must point out that he is not as good as a student with a lower mark and that a really good "B"student would be able to overcome some of these tribulations and handle the situation in a better manner than he did."

The tutor was now scraping the barrel of course and at this point the set-piece moves would take second place to the individual tactics of the different lecturers. Some of Erfert's appointees could come up with really wonderful defences of the indefensible but even the saner members would often employ unscrupulous tactics. Lady members of staff were good at bursting into tears, or fits or hysterics in order to get their own way. Older male members settled down to filibuster in the knowledge that the external examiner had a train to catch and would not be anxious to prolong the deadlock beyond certain time. Nastier types were given to implying that the examiner was motivated by racialist principles or religious bigotry. Grown men had visibly paled in the face of such accusations and had lost all stomach for a fight over their marks. But a sane and sober external examiner could still hold out and produce a trump card such as; "I do not know why the college has external examiners if they are not to have the final say over students' marks." It remained to be seen how strong and sober was Mabel Croxteth.

Dr Erfert rarely had any students of his own to supervise but when he did they rarely failed. This was partly due to his reputation and partly due to the incomprehensible way in which he defended them so that any opponent tended to retire baffled. Little habits he had such as giving out Green Shield stamps for credits and distinctions only served to increase the bewilderment. But the main weapon in the college armoury was due to his inherent good nature. His kindliness extended automatically to laying on hospitality for the external examiners which usually rendered them incapable of rational thought. Any potentially hostile visitor was not likely to get beyond his room and the contents of his drinks cupboard. Though he did not drink himself, he had unwittingly stumbled upon a remarkable defensive mechanism when he insisted on having a very full supply of Highland Malt Whisky for his visitors to sample. Externals frequently left his room uncertain of the location of the very walls of the college let alone that of the distant schools where they were to see students perform. In nine cases out of ten the hospitality rendered them harmless enough to pose no threat but some of them became rowdy and obstreperous even to the point of sitting at the back of lessons and observing in a loud stage whisper that it was all bloody rubbish.

Some insisted on taking over lessons and ended up marking themselves. Hidden but basic inclinations came out, inclinations such as childishness or kleptomania. One eminent professor was in his element helping eight year olds to measure the classroom floor whilst another one was happily stealing from the coats in the cloakroom until he returned to announce to the world that town children tended to draw cows with no udders whilst country children drew them with the necessary under part. This was promptly put to the test to the detriment of the specimen lesson to be observed.

The big trouble was that some of the externals managed to remain sane and sober throughout the whole three day period. Maybe Miss Croxteth was one of these. Sometimes their drunken colleagues could be set against them, if bribery, corruption and allegations of assault had all failed. This was one of the few things that the sane side and the crazy side of St. Brendan's agreed on. It was usually all right as long as one of the sane party was in charge of the arrangements for teaching practice but this was the year that the principal had confided in Mavis Flint that he had every confidence in her as the supremo in charge.

Mavis Flint was a tall jack-booted ex-Primary School Head teacher who had got a job in the college in answer to an advertisement for someone with experience of progressive methods. She had at that time believed passionately in "freedom." In her school she had abolished the timetable so that the teachers could be free, she had abolished playtimes so that the children could be free. She had the doors taken off their hinges so that communication (which she insisted on calling "intercourse") should be free also.

After a while, when other people were beginning to do the same sort of thing, she instinctively knew that it was time to change her views and she had become a fascist who did not believe in freedom in any of its shapes or forms. Officially she called her theory "Freedom through Regulation" but there was little of the former to be found in it. Just as people became free to fly by discovering the laws of flight, so she argued, would little children discover true freedom by being bound by more rules than either the M.C.C or the Football League had ever thought up. Nor were parents exempt. One of her more famous sayings was when addressing a parents meeting called to explain the progressive methods employed in the school, she said; "Now sit up straight and pay attention whilst I explain to you what I want you to do to help me in my work." Her one regret was that she could no longer inflict corporal punishment on children. But she saw no reason why it should not be employed in the training of student teachers.

As might be expected, she organised the teaching practice with military precision. At the briefing meeting she had maps and handouts by the dozen. She gave everyone explicit instructions about their roles and made it clear that she was not going to put up with any interference from snivelling little communist stooges. As she did so she menacingly tapped her pipe on her boot .

The plan was basically simple. A team of six examiners would stay at the college for three days and see a representative sample of students teaching in a variety of schools within a thirty mile radius. When Mr Scott had supervised the arrangements a team of six drivers undertook to get them to the various schools on time and then to ferry them elsewhere several times in the day. Mavis Flint had a team of six and a reserve team of six more, maps, iron rations, and radio communications that connected her command centre with them at all times. But she did not see to it that externals were never to see weak students or students teaching the external's own specialisms. Above all she did not see to it that Erfert's legions were kept well clear of the driving pool. She was not responsible for the geographical condition of Lancashire in winter, that land of urban jams or mists and moors, but such conditions alone would have rendered her strict timetable inoperable. So it was that in her final briefing she informed each driver of the precise distance to each school, the precise journey time that she had calculated and the times of each lesson that would be seen in each school to be visited. Most of this was lost on the motley crew in front of her. One was playing with his Rubik cube. Two were sociologists dressed identically in their uniforms of red shirts, white ties and denim tops. Long haired Art lecturers listened hard and heard nothing. A lady psychology lecturer scribbled away furiously but what she was taking down was anybody's guess.

When the great moment came the first car took off at speed. It contained a strange pair. The first was a Professor of Education recently retired and very recently inebriated, a person who exhibited some alarming characteristics. Almost his first act upon entering the car was to steal the knob from the gear stick and to attempt to eat it. Then he had a go at most of the switches in an apparent attempt to prize them away from the fascia but achieved more success with the tax disc displayed on the window in front of him.

His companion, though quite sober, was perhaps the more dangerous of the two. He was in no way put out by the professor's strange behaviour nor was he in the least perturbed by the complicated instructions given to him by Mavis Flint. He had forgotten them anyway. He was a sculptor by profession and thought of little else than getting back to his latest creation which was an arrangement of household bricks to represent the Crucifixion. So Mavis was disturbed to find that soon after setting off down the drive he had turned the wrong way to get to Oswaldtwistle where his first school lay. She assured herself that he must be making a detour to buy cigarettes. But he was not going to buy cigarettes. He was tootling along quite happily observing the Professor's attempts to eat the tax disc. This was still absorbing him when he ran into the back of the bus and had to face not only an irate bus driver but also an inquisitive policeman who found it difficult to believe that he was on his way to Oswaldtwistle, which was in the other direction, and that the distinguished academic beside him had only just that minute eaten the tax disc of the vehicle.

The second and third vehicles seemed to set off in the right directions for their respective destinations but the fourth car shot off like a bullet in the general direction of Oswaldtwistle instead of Manchester. In the car was a sociologist from St. Brendan's and an external examiner who was a committed disciple of Dr.Erfert. They were engaged in an animated conversation about the sociological implications of one of the external's favourite theories. He did not believe in the current system of teacher training and preferred a system derived from that of driving licences. This involved the giving of a teaching certificate to every student upon their entry to college and the endorsing of it from time to time if the student failed to live up to any of the expectations implied.

"Wouldn't it be better to treat it as a bus ticket?" suggested the sociologist. "Then you could clip holes in it for every weakness or misdemeanour and so the physical size of the ticket would diminish before the very eyes of the student until it no longer guaranteed qualified teacher status because those words would no longer appear on it."

The external examiner thought that a capital idea and then tried to extend it so that it embraced all sorts of solutions for elitism, racism, exam nerves and the socio-economic advantages enjoyed by the middle class.

"We could even extend it to Adult education," he proclaimed in triumph. "We could give every single adult in the country such a ticket, though many of them would lose it I fear. Then everyone would be able to teach everyone else, officially as it were, until they proved unsuitable for the task."

"Yes," shouted his companion excitedly. "And don't forget parents. Possession of such a certificate would be a great step towards intelligent parenthood. All parents could be required to have one before they brought up children."

"Before they conceived children," corrected his companion.

The conversation was proving so interesting to them that they were quite oblivious to their surroundings and they spent an hour or so speeding up and down the motorway stretch between Manchester and Burnley whilst they refined their idea and agreed on the co-authorship of an article for the educational press. Then they adjourned to a pub to write it. In the early afternoon they reported by radio to Mavis that they had visited two startled students in Oswaldtwistle who had been totally unprepared for their unscheduled visit that day.

Car number five was doing quite nicely until it too reported to Mavis that it also had arrived at Oswaldtwistle and had visited a few students not on the official list. But it was car number six that carried the danger woman. For an H.M.I. she appeared to be remarkably sane and sober, and had enough of the "real" world about her to turn up on time and to expect the driver to be on time also. She had enough road sense to guide the driver along the right route and enough common sense to ignore his babbling. She was so efficient that she turned up early to see Dave teaching his English lesson to Junior Four and caught instead his lesson on History with Junior Three, a lesson for which he was totally unprepared and it showed.

"Pay attention everyone," he began. "Open your books at page ten."

"We haven't got any books sir," was the inevitable reply.

There was a pause whilst the books were tracked down and he was dismayed to see the lady writing copious notes at the back of the room.

"Did anyone see the film about the Vikings on Tele the other night?" he asked hopefully.

"Sir that wasn't about the Vikings. It was about Attila the Hun"" said one little smart Alec.

"No, that must have been another film. I was watching myself last night," lied Dave. He quietened the chorus of protests and was relieved to see a little hand go up.

"Please sir, was there really an Old King Cole?"

"No," said Dave.

"Who was the Black Prince then sir?"

""Never mind."

He then decided to cut his losses.

"Now you all have your books. Open them at page ten and you will see a picture of a Viking ship or Longboat. I want you to draw it for me and to colour it in. The crayons are at the front."

He knew as soon as he said it that his command would have disastrous results. There was a dull roar as the chairs were pushed back and everyone made a rush to the front to grab the best crayons.

"Get back, Get back," shouted Dave in desperation as he fought manfully to get them all seated again. The lady scribbling away at the back, now had a fair sized novel in front of her.

At the end of the lesson she came up to him and informed him that she was sorry but she could not pass him on that performance and Dave could only agree with her.

That night he took his troubles to Mr Scott who received the news by clicking his tongue in annoyance. He knew that others far worse than Dave were actually getting away with murder.

"Leave it to me," he advised. Then he added mysteriously; "There is more than one way to skin a rabbit. We must fight fire with fire." Dave was very crest-fallen. He had long since given up hope of ever showing up Erfert but now he would have only the credibility of a failed student to back up any criticisms he might make.

When the afternoon of the big meeting came the students were all on edge. They knew only too well that their futures were in the hands of some very doubtful people although they had reason to believe that they would be on the side of the students in any confrontation with external examiners. Everything that could be done had been done, by sane and loony members of staff alike. One of the external examiners was missing because he was in police hands. One had to miss the meeting in order to catch the last train to Cardiff which, he was unreliably informed, went very early in the afternoon. Two were more than a little drunk and one was an Erfertian disciple. There remained the one real problem, the lady who had observed Dave's disastrous lesson. Not only was she under instructions to fail him but he was eminently deserving of being failed. She had survived the nervous shock brought on by two obscene phone calls that morning and she was putting up a spirited defence of her proposal to fail him when Mr Scott produced his trump card.

Mr Scott produced a weapon so secret that many of the staff had never seen it used before. He called upon the resident Chinese gentleman to defend Dave. He had never actually met Dave but that did not matter because he defended him with very great vigour and great skill that was unappreciated because what he said was completely unintelligible to the assembled academics. They cheered him none the less at what seemed to be appropriate moments and he beamed his pleasure as he launched into more and more arguments. Even MacPudding was moved to stand on his feet to support him in an even more unintelligible manner. The lady was visibly sagging but still held to her guns until a little note was pushed across the table to her from the Principal himself. Written on it was the simple message; "It might be as well for you to return to London. The D.E.S. has just announced the privatisation of the Inspectorate with many job cuts."

"The swines," was her only muttered comment as she decided to let Smith pass as the only act of revenge that she could think of for the treachery of the D.E.S.

The double oak doors of the conference room swung open and the hordes of students who had just happened to be waiting nonchalantly outside were given the first intimation that yet again St. Brendan's had achieved a hundred percent pass rate. They could now practise their 'skills'on other people's children, their own being sent to private schools if possible. They had achieved a measure of social respectability for which their training had hardly equipped them. Even Dave's problems had been solved. He could teach if he wanted to. He could get married if he wanted to. He could denounce his college if he wanted to without being labelled as a malcontented failure. But first there were the examinations to contend with.

Chapter 26

The examinations were not too bad in themselves. It was the examiners that had to be watched. When the Academic Board convened itself as the Examinations Panel anything could happen. The Head of Publicity and Merchandising whose main task was to sell T Shirts with the College Logo printed on, informed the Academic Board with great solemnity that the College must change or go under. They must compete, they must challenge, they must be competitive, they must win.

Somewhat exhausted by his unaccustomed bout of oratory he subsided into his chair before he had to answer the few members who wanted to know why they must fight, compete, challenge, win or indeed, why they must change anything at all. To him it was all so simple; change was imperative and its advantages self evident. Only the blindest of the blind could not see it his way so it did not need to be proved, only implemented. Otherwise, he further informed them, "we will be dead in the water". Unfortunately his arrival at St. Brendan's had coincided with one of Erfert's moments of infatuation with "Change-As-A-Categorical-Imperative" and so he had found a receptive ear at the top.

Within a week the two of them had conspired to change the very name of the college to indicate a close relationship with the local community and to knock down the lovely high sandstone walls in order to invite in the local community and encourage a mix of town and gown. This mix took the form of gangs of motor-cycle youths who were only too anxious to mix it with the gowns of "No Hopers" as they called the students and whose boisterous contribution to the rich mixture caused the walls to be rebuilt at the request of the local constabulary.

"I think that I am right in saying that when we mark our students we *still*," (he lingered on the word as if to emphasise the stupidity of the practice), "we still give 60% of the marks for examination work and 40% for course work."

The wise ones nodded their assent to this statement of their practice and the crazy ones were already starting to shout "Outrageous" on principle. On which encouragement he further ventured to propose that the 40% should be broken up into smaller elements to include for instance, oral contributions to seminars or, as he put it, 'OCS'.

"Won't that be difficult to handle?", asked Mr Scott.

"Not the way I plan to handle it", replied Loo. "All students will be required to speak in lectures or seminars and all other occasions of tuition, and their contributions will be marked and used to form part of their examination marks".

This masterpiece of non-explanation failed to impress Mr Scott and he pressed on with his question. "But how can you handle up to thirty students all making an oral contribution at some length? It would take up all the teaching time just to administer the oral test."

"I am bound to say that if every time somebody suggests some new, constructive change you are going to reply with negative, destructive criticism of that kind then it is a waste of our time having any meetings at all," was the only reply that he got or was ever likely to get. But he pressed on.

"How could you ensure that all the students are treated fairly? Some are shy and get tongue-tied; some gabble on but have nothing worthwhile to say; some will have disabilities; some will just be absent on their particular day. I must tell you that I do not think that it is a practical proposition."

But he had already lost the fight because, although Peter Loo had nothing relevant to say there were plenty of others round the table who had suggestions to make.

"I resent the slur that you have made on the professional integrity of my colleagues," boomed the Amendment-in-Search-of- A-Resolution. "I have every confidence that complete objectivity will be maintained."

"I concur," said the Head of Quality Assurance. "All that is needed is for us to fail anyone who is away and to video tape all the contributions so that they can be shown to a another lecturer and be second marked by him - or her," he hastily added.

"Yes," said the Head of Inter-Personal Relationships, who normally never spoke to anyone. "I think that they could also be transcribed and printed out in hard copy so that a third person can adjudicate between the first two markers. We would have to do this anyway for the deaf or dumb or the deaf and dumb students. We must treat them all equally. As for absentees; they would of course fail."

"We would need another hard copy for the external examiner anyway. We could hardly expect him to sit through sessions over thirty two weeks in the year just to wait for an oral contribution from every student," remarked Mr Scott with what he thought was obvious irony. It was lost on his colleagues however.

"Why not?" went up the roar which was then followed by an attack on lazy, unreasonable external examiners whose only aim in life was to obstruct necessary change. Change by this time had become transmuted into "Progress" which made the externals even more unreasonable.

"Could I say something?" stammered Dave only to be shouted down and told that a student had nothing to contribute on matters relating to oral contributions of students.

Sometime later he was glad of his rejection because it exonerated him from charges of complicity when the campus was filled with hordes of lecturers carrying notebooks, tape recorders, video recorders, concealed as well as openly displayed, eavesdropping on conversations and making mysterious entries about what was said. Mr Scott made a little note at the Board to remind himself as Examinations Officer that the final formula for arriving at marks was to remain in the hands of the College Examinations Officer so he was not really worried about the outcome. He merely ventured to suggest that a ventriloquist might be employed to help particularly bad failures. He was not altogether surprised to find that his suggestion found favour with some of his colleagues.

He got Dave through the examination by taking every mark he had ever gained at any stage and rounding up all the decimals until they exceeded the pass mark. But Dave never knew that.

Chapter 27

After his rather unconventional proposal in the confessional of St. Francis's Church, Dave's life had changed appreciably. He had learned to be more tolerant of members of staff and he had reason to be grateful to the system he had despised, for saving him from ignominy. Although he tried from time to time to work up a lather of indignation, he was slowly but surely being sucked into the system itself.

"After all," Jane pointed out, "everyone else accepts it. Why can't you?"

But there is something about Yorkshire men that prevents them from accepting things, and there was something deep within him that constantly urged him to rebel against such a barmy system. That he did accept in the end was due to the influence of a most unlikely person. His conversion came as a consequence of his receiving instructions in the Catholic Faith in order to marry Jane. He was never to join her Faith as such but he did receive an insight into a world in which people like Erfert could flourish and he received it from the crippled Fr.Terence.

Quite apart from the various religious propositions that were explained to him he was deeply impressed by this simple friar, confined to a wheel chair and helping others when he ought to have been permanently looked after himself. Dave was staggered by the sight of him literally dragging himself to the altar for his daily mass and was tremendously moved by the obvious way in which he *was* what he wanted others to be. He was the opposite of everything that was phoney in the world of Erfert. The thing that impressed Dave most of all was that this simple man could have held his own in any institution of learning in the country. There was no sign on the notice-board to say that Fr. Terence O.F.M. held a double doctorate, from Cambridge and from the Gregorian University in Rome. His quality came from his advice not from his ornaments.

"It took you a long time to tell me you were an academic," Dave reproached him one day.

"I am not," said the priest.

"You have got more qualifications than most of our staff."

"Qualifications don't make academics, I think. Anyway, I am a priest not an academic as such."

"I bet you don't believe me about what goes on in my academic world," persisted Dave.

"I have no reason to disbelieve you. My own academic background was a bit different of course. A lot of my studies took place on the continent and through the medium of Latin and in a more Christian context."

Dave took in a sharp intake of breath. Here was a man who had studied Theology to a high degree, through the medium of Latin, in an environment of Italian and on top of a Cambridge doctorate. He had mastered as incidentals things that Erfert's staff would have been proud to flaunt as their greatest achievement! And yet it had to be prized out of him because his immediate task was to help Dave understand a few piddling bits and pieces of religion in order to marry Jane in a Catholic Church.

"I know that you are not a fit man, and don't get me wrong, but couldn't the Church find you something more high-powered to do than this?"

"That may be the difference between you and me, and between Erfert and me. To me there is nothing more important than being a priest and there is nothing more important than a priest's work. Any academic study that I may have done is to equip me in that work, not the other way round. Scholars might like to act as if they are omniscient, and their disciplines might attempt to explain the world but they are God's creatures none the less and their disciplines need explaining themselves."

Dave was getting a bit out of his depth at this point and changed the subject. Even at sport, the young Fr.Terence had excelled everyone he had ever met. Jane supplied the information that the priest had been a handsome, All-Ireland international greatly admired by the girls in his Mayo county. There had been many a broken heart when he had announced a higher calling. The priest laughed this off in a slightly embarrassed way.

"May I ask what happened to you. When did you become ill?"

"It only goes to show that you cannot count on things like health. I was perfectly all right and had just finished saying mass in my last parish when I stumbled and fell as I left the altar. Over the next few days I stumbled a few more times and consulted a doctor. He eventually told me that I had Motor-Neuron Disease and would become more clumsy and awkward as time went by. When I could not cope without a wheel-chair they sent me here because it is easier."

"They sent you here?"

"The order sent me. That is the way it goes in religious orders. You do as you are told and go where you are sent."

Dave found it difficult to get his mind round that. An eminent academic, doing menial work, becoming incapable, and being sent to eke out a pain-wracked existence as a miserable non-entity in an obscure little parish. The contrast was all the more stark because that parish was full of overrated so-called academics who were not fit to be in the same room as this man.

"But enough about me. Listen, I want to get you two safely married off within the next six months and I want to perform the ceremony myself. That is if you have no objection."

"I have no objection. But I don't see what all the hurry is," said Dave with his typical Yorkshire stubbornness.

"I am afraid that is all the time he has left to live," Jane informed him.

Dave was stunned by this seemingly casual remark but neither of the two Catholics seemed to be the least put out by the thought of death.

"Don't worry about my feelings," said Fr.Terence. "I have no fear of death. It comes to all of us. That is what my priesthood is all about. And that my lad is what your education is all about or should be. Your Education lectures will no doubt have taught you that schooling is all about educating people for Life. The trouble is that people differ about what Life is. Life to me is about preparing for the next Life. So education is really not just about this world but also about the next and my degrees which seem to impress you have equipped me to face that prospect not just to give me a bit of one-upmanship. Life is about Death. Think about it and I am sure you will see something in it."

"It seems a bit morbid to me," grumbled Dave. "And I don't quite see how that explains the lunacies that go on in the world of education. Your not saying that they all should be Catholics?"

"No, of course not. But I come from a slightly different academic tradition remember. Call it the broader European tradition if you like. If Education is for Life and Life is for Death then any education that is divorced from man and his ultimate destiny is *deracine*, so to speak."

"It sounds fine, but in practice, I am in an institution of higher education and I seem to be surrounded by a bunch of loonies, some of them highly qualified, pursuing their own disciplines without much reference to any other discipline and certainly without any obvious relevance to man or his destiny whether it be a religious or an atheistic one.

I am afraid that that is one of the problems of our age and of teacher training in particular. I am sure they instil into you the maxim that you must have an aim. Only in relation to an aim can you devise appropriate methods and syllabi. Only in relation to an aim can you be successful, or fail for that matter. You are not the first to discover that they do not practise what they preach. I will bet that your

Education lectures consist of separate disciplines of Philosophy, Psychology, Sociology and the rest which seem unconnected to the point where you wonder whether there is any such thing as Education as a subject at all."

Dave nodded. He was now beginning to see some light at the end of the tunnel.

"Well I belong to the older school which says that you have an end in view when you set out to educate someone, be that someone a pupil or a student teacher. If you happen to think that religion is irrelevant to this life and the next then of course you can pursue some other end but to my mind a lot of people have not replaced religion with anything else so they pursue their psychology, or their sociology as ends in themselves or as explanatory disciplines for the whole of the world phenomena, forgetting that they are themselves only part of the greater picture. When you distort things in that way you achieve a kind of madness. It is not so much that they are insane but they have a distorted view of things and it can look like the same thing."

"Well Erfert is religious in his own way but he certainly tends to distort things by interpreting everything from the point of view of a couple of educational disciplines."

"It is a great pity that he never seems to have read Newman on the real nature of Knowledge. Have you come across Newman on the Idea of a University?"

Dave hadn't of course.

"He more or less says that all knowledge should add up. If the world is in a constant state of flux and chaos then of course, nothing will add up, but if there is a creator who made it all and who has a plan, then it should add up. We tend to study reality from the standpoint of our respective disciplines and become experts in bits of knowledge and in bits of specialisms but we should not assume that those fragments explain the whole picture. You can have highly educated nonsense and academically respectable nonsense for that very reason. At one time Theology was regarded as the Queen of the Sciences because it gave a context for all the other disciplines. Now other things rush in to fill the vacuum. In a general sort of way Science is the Queen now. But in practice that means a lot of separate sciences vie with each other for the privilege of providing some overall explanatory principle for reality. A lop-sided scientist may have lots of valuable things to tell us but he is not in a position to explain the world to us and he should not try. He is like a man studying an eye on a laboratory bench. He may know all there is to know about the eye, its texture, its physics, its defects etc. But he must also know the eye in its context i.e. in the face. Unless he has the whole picture he does not know the eye or the face."

"Are you saying that we cannot know anything unless we know everything? And isn't that impossible?"

"I suppose I am saying that in a way. Obviously I am not saying that Heaven is only for brain boxes and that everyone has to study everything to the nth degree. But I think that what we lack now is a context into which we can place the knowledge that we accumulate. All the X-Rays and photographs and measurements in the world will not explain the eye if it just lies there on the plate but if we know its context we know it better. In one sense it is the addition sum of all the different sciences that study the eye and in one sense it is a grand vision that comes first and gives all these other disciplines some meaning and purpose. I have a religious grand vision. Others will have different explanatory principles. I feel sorry for the people who have no vision and no principles at all. If all is chaos and anarchy there is no point in studying things in their context because there is no context. The specialist can then elevate his specialism into some sort of explanatory principle rather than a descriptive discipline and there is no one to gainsay him. A psychologist might kid himself that he can explain all there is to know about a man. But a sociologist might make the same claim, a social-psychologist might feel in a superior position to both. To a Christian all these sciences are but helps towards understanding man. They provide no complete explanations in themselves and to kid yourself otherwise is a form of madness although the world would not recognise it as such and would indeed reward them for their academic efforts. I would not blame Erfert so much for his apparent madness but the society that produced him and promoted him. When you can change that society you will unseat him and not before. One thing is clear. I will not live to see it. Nor will you I suspect."

Chapter 28

Having overcome the main obstacle, the teaching practice, the students of St. Brendan's could take it easy for a while. They had to face the examinations, of course, but these were in the capable hands of Mr Scott and provided no more than the normal hazards of student life. Much more important was the finding of a good job in the teaching profession. This required early application and the submission of a testimonial and two references. As they were often competing against each other for the best jobs there was a limit to the camaraderie that could be expected. It was customary to get a testimonial from the Principal and the references from lecturers who knew them well. Some tutors wrote the truth and so did irreparable harm to the student's chances. Some wrote manifest lies and were equally useless. Some wrote just the right blend of truth and falsehood that impressed would-be employers. These were worth cultivating.

The testimonial from the Principal was usually good for a laugh but then was thrown away in favour of one written by Mr Scott. The reason for this went back to the principal's antipathy to references and testimonials. It was his view that such documents were useless because they were written by people who actually knew the student. Such persons could not possibly be objective. Moreover, a student was only likely to approach a person who would speak well of him. His own view, expressed at the time of his arrival at the college and considered at that time to be an example of his delicious wit, was that they should be written by persons who had no knowledge of the student but he had since come to a compromise with the saner members of staff. The official system was that he would sign a testimonial that had been drawn up by a senior member of staff who in turn would base his remarks on material submitted by people who knew the student personally.

All perhaps would have been well if the senior member of staff who wrote the testimonial had not been one of his appointees, Brenda Ottaway, lecturer in Drama, part-time mystic, and semi-pro astrologer. Her Drama lecturers were little better than the Witches of Pendle set to music and the welcome to the college of real witches to play the appropriate parts. It was a surprise choice when she got the job of Senior Lecturer (Pastoral) in charge of student records and references, but it enabled her to indulge her passion of forecasting people's futures. She tended to throw away all the evidence that accumulated in her office and relied instead upon her own deep reflection as she perused photographs of the students and studied their birth dates and star sign in her permanently darkened room. Curiously enough she was often quite accurate about the students concerned.

Around about the time of the mid-term break in the last term of his course, Dave, like others, received the message that his testimonial was ready for collection. He did not hurry to collect what he knew would be a worthless document even if it truly reflected his ability as a teacher. He was interested in Martin Lockett's however as his friends were comparing theirs.

"Like all Cancerians, Mr Lockett is a great worrier and tends to keep his worries bottled up inside of him. If he could relax more he could become a much more effective teacher than he is at the moment."

Jane was promised good luck in financial and in matrimonial matters and was not unwilling to wave the testimonial in front of Dave as confirmation that she was a good catch.

Alun Evans was described as a sensitive soul. "Whilst some people might find his ideas impractical, he should not be put off by their opposition. It is not recommended that he be asked to teach any Librans."

Eventually Dave summoned up enough enthusiasm to go to the principal's house to collect his own. A stupid astrological prediction would only lend weight to his dossier on Erfert, although that dossier no longer took up much of his time or attention. He was a little worried that it might not be an astrological testimonial at all. One that stemmed from young Brian might be worse in view of Dave's assault on him with the cane and his later career in crime.

He was still musing on this prospect when he was overtaken by a middle-aged woman who was being dragged along by a large Alsatian dog which seemed determined to get into the Guinness Book of Records. As she whizzed past, she shouted out a request for directions to the Principal's house but hardly had Dave raised his arm to point out the way when the dog was bounding up the drive of that very residence, overtaking as it did so a group of young local urchins who were dragging behind them two or three dogs of dubious pedigree. As Dave got nearer to the door he found himself at the end of a long queue of such animals as one might find outside the P.D.S.A. dispensary. The dogs were running all over the garden, fretting and fighting and performing all sorts of unmentionable but biologically necessary duties.

With his back to the front door, clutching several letters and papers, and besieged by a throng of noisy dogs and shouting people was the Principal himself. He was beaming happily as he always did when one of his experiments was a great success, but he was in great danger of being crushed against the house wall until Dave pushed him through the open door leaving some of the dogs to eat the letters he had held in his hand.

"Well, is it or isn't it?" demanded a large woman in a leather coat.

"I very much regret that it is not," he replied with exquisite and genuine charm.

"How can it be?" shouted another woman.. "When it is this one that I have brought. Look it knows him. It is licking his face."

"I am afraid that it is not that one either," he insisted from between the legs of several affectionate animals just as Dave helped him to his feet. "In fact none of these dogs is the one I am looking for."

At this point the crowd looked as if it would turn quite ugly but Erfert, as usual, got out of it by his good manners.

"I must express to you all my gratitude for your help and the trouble you have taken in bringing all these dogs to my home for me to see. I am only sorry that your efforts have not borne fruit on this occasion. As some small recompense perhaps you would all like to enter my house and take tea and biscuits with me and my wife, and this

244

young man. My wife will be delighted to meet you. Bring the dogs in as well."

Dave could see by his wife's face that the Principal's words were probably just that little bit optimistic so he offered to assist her in the kitchen whilst Erfert continued to address the multitude. He had in his hand an envelope rescued from the dog and the dirt. It had his name on it and he stood for a while reading it whilst Mrs Erfert put the kettle on.

"To whom it may concern," it began. "I understand that Mr David Smith is shortly to apply for a post in your employment. I should like to recommend him to you. He was born under the sign of Leo so he should be an excellent prospect for any position that you might have available in the summer months. According to the information that we have available at the moment his life is due to enter a new and exciting phase but he must not be tempted to relax or many of the gains made might be lost. A home or property matter needs to be settled in the next month or two and then he can look forward to a rewarding career, if not in teaching, in something to do with meeting people. You might like to know that his lucky colour is red and his lucky number is eight."

"Oh dear," she said. "I see that you have got your report."

"Not that it will do me much good," grumbled Dave.

"If I were you I should give it back to the Alsatian to finish off." And with that she grabbed it out of his hand and tossed it through the window to the Alsatian which greedily gobbled it up.

Dave was surprised by the first public act of disloyalty that he had seen from her in all the years he had spent at the college. It seems that she was in a bad mood because of the invasion of the house by the canine league of friends. She explained what it was all about.

"It is all part of my husband's plan to bring town and gown closer together and to combine it with a sociological experiment. He is using a technique which proved successful a few years ago. In order to break the ice with strangers, especially those that he wanted to interview without their knowing it, he would go up to them and claim that he had lost his dog and asking them if they had, by any chance, seen it. If they asked what kind of dog, he would describe the first kind of dog that came into his mind. People rather take to him you know and there is never any shortage of people willing to help him find his dog. Little boys have been turning up here all week with a vast assortment of dogs that they must have kidnapped in order to claim a reward. His search for his dog reached the newspaper and the phone has never stopped ringing since. A dog hunt has been organised on a grand scale. No dog is safe. You just happened to arrive with the first batch of the day. To be honest I am not very pleased."

"Don't you every feel embarrassed by his goings on?" Dave was bold enough to ask.

"I used to be. He does get some silly ideas from time to time. But don't judge him too harshly. He means well and these people will all leave here loving him, I do assure you. Wait until you hear his reception at the Going-Down Dinner and you will see why your mission here never had a chance of success. He is invincible even if he is a little odd at times. By the way, I have not forgotten how you helped young

Brian that night when you baby-sat for us. Don't worry about the testimonial. I will write a good one for you myself and get my husband to sign it."

Chapter 29

The Going-Down Dinner was the highlight of the year. Nostalgia set in early. The students were dressed smartly for the first and last time in some cases. The staff reverted to type. Miriam Woodstock volunteered for cloakroom duty so that she would not have to meet anyone in conversation. Mathew Brown was checking the tickets and Mavis Flint was organising the buffet with an iron discipline. Mrs Mason was graciously greeting people as they arrived because it gave her the chance to inspect their heads.

The Dinner was nothing to write home about but throughout it the noise level rose as a testimony to the fact that everyone was enjoying it. Then came the speeches. Macpudding began the proceedings with an impassioned but regrettably incoherent diatribe against the Yellow Peril that was threatening the western world. Then came Mr Scott with a predictably witty yet cynical contribution.

"I must congratulate all you ladies and gentlemen for having had the ingenuity to outwit the examiners in the most shameless fashion," he said. "I trust that you will leave us all the more refreshed for your period of convalescence here and that you will hesitate before mentioning us when you tell people about your training for the teaching profession. If you do care to remember us from time to time when you are out in the big wide world earning vast sums of money you might also care to remember this last piece of advice which I give you free. The educational process is like the steady drip drip drip of rain water on the window pane. As it dries it leaves a tiny deposit of dirt upon the surface of that pane. Other small deposits accumulate and build up imperceptibly into something of weight and substance. That pane, ladies and gentlemen is the DIRTY LITTLE MIND OF THE AVERAGE CHILD (pause for laugh) and YOU ARE THE DRIPS WHO WILL PERFORM THIS MINOR MIRACLE (pause for longer and final laugh). The problem is that some drips never seem to dry up when they ought to."

He sat down to great applause and then it was the turn of the Principal. Dave expected him to announce some lunatic new policy for the coming year or that he just received an honour from the Queen or some such nonsense. But it was a different Dr. Erfert who good naturedly acknowledged the cat-calls as he stood up to speak.

His words were simple enough, chosen with care and delivered with great sincerity. He assured them that it was a great pleasure for him and his wife to attend this function and to see the product of three years hard work on everyone's part come to fruition. He recalled their entry as raw recruits, their first efforts at teaching and the efforts of the staff to improve them; he praised their hard work and the support of their families and he expressed his hopes that they would go on to bigger and better things.

Teaching, he reminded them, was a noble profession. It demanded dedication. What could be more responsible than to be entrusted with the malleable young minds of the next generation? What could be more gratifying than to know that you have played a part in influencing the physical intellectual and moral development of a young person? He then quoted a small published verse, well known in Catholic circles, which he said he had been given by a local priest, sadly no longer with us. It was to stick in the minds of his audience for many years to come.

"I took a piece of plastic clay,
And gently fashioned it one day.
And as my fingers pressed it, still,
It moved and yielded to my will.
I came again when days were past;
That piece of clay was hard at last.
It still my early impress bore,
But I could change that shape no more.
I took a piece of living clay
And gently moulded it one day
I moulded it with skill and art
A young child's soft and yielding heart.
I came again when days were gone,
It was a man I gazed upon.
He still my early imprint bore,
But I could change that shape no more."

Somehow the Principal had the knack of reaching the heart strings of his audience. Most of the ladies were now crying and some of the men were very close to tears, even rough necked rugby players. It stemmed from the niceness of the man, from his goodness and his sincerity from his simplicity and his genuine liking for his students. His wife sat proudly by his side in the knowledge that his eccentricities would all be forgiven by the students who would never forget him.

He had finished and had sat down for some time before the audience realised it and burst into first a ripple of applause and then a riot of clapping and cheering whilst he sat blinking behind his spectacles and sipping his orange juice which had been his sole refreshment throughout the whole evening.

All this left Dave almost as confused as ever. He had long since given up all hope of denouncing Erfert and all intention of harming him but he still could not reconcile the fact that the imparter of the speech could also hold such idiotic schemes in the same brain. He was all the more confused when he went to the bar and found himself standing next to Erfert and one of Erfert's more unfortunate appointees. He was explaining some of the changes that he intended to make in the college next year to this adoring disciple.

It was all about distractions to study in a world dominated by pop-culture. How could anyone study when Top of the Pops was blaring out from the television set? The answer was to turn the college into a place of pop culture and to have music blaring out all day so that work would become the welcome distraction. If the students approached this distraction with the same enthusiasm they showed for other distractions the college was on to a winner. The D.E.S. should be informed at once.

The mention of the D.E.S. jerked Dave back to his own rather precarious situation vis a vis his employers. Was he to go back? He was not aware that they were plotting against him of course but he certainly knew that he was not the flavour of the month at headquarters. Then he thought of Jane, his wife of a few weeks. And he thought of Fr.Terence whose last priestly act had been the marriage ceremony. He had died a happy man despite his cruel illness. He had died a simple friar not a double doctor. He had made his mark and left his message in an ordinary waiting room not a packed lecture theatre. He had given Dave a glimmer of an understanding of a mad world that promoted mad things because they were propounded by "experts" who had no wider vision than their own limited expertise. Their discipline was their God and their methodology was their end. He could either rebel in his customary fruitless search for integrity or he could accept the rules of the game as everyone else seemed to do.

He made up his mind, grabbed Jane, rushed home and wrote a letter to his employers at the D.E.S which included his best judgement on the matter.

"I am now in a position to answer the question which caused me to be sent to this college in the first place. I am pleased to be able to confirm that Dr. Erfert is without doubt a genius. His presence here is an undeniable inspiration to all who are fortunate enough to study under him. Your own original estimate of his worth was unerringly accurate and my own incredibly naive.

"On the vexed question of Emolumentally Lucrative Regressive Disincentives, may I confess that I misinterpreted the line which referred to 'saturated job satisfaction in anything other than a dysfunctioning occupational environment'? I took it to mean that a super-saturated job satisfaction was to increase in inverse proportion to the injection of the regressive disincentive, whereas I now realise that the dysfunctioning occupational environment would introduce a relatively static variable which would compensate for the multilateral retardation effect.

"I further realise that such an explanation must have been apparent to you all along. I can only apologise for having doubted your estimation of the great man and his theories. I have now learned my lesson and would ask only one favour of you. Would you please release me from my position in the department so that I can seek a teaching post in this area? I hope thereby to keep in contact with Dr.Erfert and so deepen my understanding of both Education and Human Nature."

Theophilus the cat opened the letter, accepted the resignation and purred. Some would be forgiven for thinking that the animal sneered.